Redefining Prostate Cancer

Why One Size Does Not Fit All

Steven Lamm, MD, Herbert Lepor, MD,
and Dan Sperling, MD

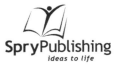

SpryPublishing
ideas to life

This edition is published by
Spry Publishing LLC
2500 South State Street
Ann Arbor, MI 48104 USA

Printed and bound in the United States of America.

10   9   8   7   6   5   4   3   2

Library of Congress Control Number: 2013937938

Paperback ISBN: 978-1-938170-31-7
eBook ISBN: 978-1-938170-32-4

Illustrations by Robin Hite

Privacy: Some names and identifying details have been changed to protect
the privacy of individuals.

To my father, Dr. Arnold Lam, who impressed upon me that "one size does not fit all" when treating patients. —SL

To my wife, Ellen Shapiro, MD, who over the past 31 years has been my best friend as we navigated our personal and professional lives together, and to my exceptionally talented and wonderful children, Abbey and Lauren, who one day may take over for Mommy and Daddy practicing the art and noble profession of medicine. —HL

To my father and mother, Dr. Arnold and Joyce Sperling, my wife Eve, and sons Ryan and Evan for all their love, support, and guidance, and to the patients whom I have been privileged to meet and who have inspired me to dedicate myself to fighting prostate cancer. —DS

Contents

Introduction

In 2011, the U.S. Preventive Services Task Force (USPSTF)—an independent organization of medical experts in disease prevention and evidence-based medicine—issued new recommendations on prostate cancer screening that threw the world of urology and men's health into a tailspin. After examining all the available clinical research, the USPSTF reversed previous recommendations for prostate-specific antigen (PSA) prostate cancer screening. The organization stated that utilizing the PSA test resulted in little to no improvement in the prostate cancer death rate, while at the same time carrying with it a large percentage of false-positive results that were responsible for unnecessary and potentially harmful evaluation and treatments in many men. In short, universal PSA screening was doing more harm than good.

On the face of it, this recommendation is understandable. PSA screening is an imperfect test, known for a wide margin of false-positive and false-negative results. Many diagnostic and treatment procedures for prostate cancer result in erectile dysfunction, incontinence, and other health problems. Better screening tests are certainly needed, and researchers continue to seek out new, more reliable markers for prostate cancer detection and risk stratification.

But at the same time, the cold hard facts are that PSA screening is currently the best widely available test we have at our disposal for early detection of prostate cancer and PSA screening has resulted in a

40% decline in the death rate from prostate cancer. If we abandon the PSA screening test for men over 50, what can we do to detect the most common cancer in men that kills an American male every eight minutes? Should we summarily disregard this test for all men recognizing that many lives are saved by early detection and curative intervention?

The most sensible answer seems to be to get smarter about how we apply the PSA test. An active 55-year-old man who has a strong family history of prostate cancer is likely a better candidate for PSA screening than a frail 85-year-old. While we wait for a better gold standard test, we should not hold back from using PSA screening for men who can benefit from it. If you are a patient, you deserve a say in this decision. Have a discussion with your doctor about the pros and cons of PSA testing in your particular situation.

We are also living in an exciting time for prostate cancer diagnosis and treatment. As you'll read in this book, there are promising and innovative new techniques for evaluating and treating cancer in the prostate that may control the disease while avoiding many of the grievous side effects.

The three of us come from very different areas of medicine. Dr. Lamm is an internist and men's health specialist who meets men at the beginning of their prostate cancer journey. Dr. Lepor is a leading urologist and researcher who codeveloped the nerve-sparing radical prostatectomy and has performed thousands of prostate cancer surgeries. And Dr. Sperling is an interventional radiologist specializing in advanced imaging techniques for the prostate and cutting-edge new forms of minimally invasive treatment. We have found that, by working together, we can offer our patients a collaborative care approach that results in the best individual treatment for them.

Above all, we recognize that just as every prostate cancer is different, every man who receives this diagnosis has very different needs and expectations. Age, medical history, family situation, occupation, emotional needs—all of these are factors in finding the treatment approach that is right for you. What is a good choice for one man may be completely wrong for another, even if they have a very similar type and grade of prostate cancer. "One size fits all" treatments are the past, not the future, of prostate cancer care.

We have written *Redefining Prostate Cancer* with this in mind. In these pages, men and their loved ones will find answers to their prostate cancer questions, from diagnosis through treatment and beyond. It is the most up-to-date review on genetic markers for risk stratification, imaging, and focal therapy currently available for prostate cancer patients. And through the stories of patients just like you, you'll learn how men from all walks of life have found health and improved quality of life in the course of their prostate cancer journey.

CHAPTER ONE

Your Prostate: An Owner's Guide

One Man's Story

John is a 58-year-old man who hasn't been inside a doctor's office in more than 15 years. His wife Denise made an appointment for him with Dr. Lamm for a routine physical and he agreed, although he "feels fine." A little tired, sure, but he's not as young as he used to be. And, he works long hours at a demanding job and can't always get enough sleep. He's mainly visiting the doctor to set his wife's mind at rest.

For her part, Denise worries that her husband may not be as healthy as he seems to think he is. As they start planning for his up-coming early retirement, she's finally gotten him to agree to a checkup just to make sure everything is working right. She's also noticed that John tires easily and isn't as interested in sex as he used to be. Denise worries that his lack of stamina could be a sign of a health problem, a thought she doesn't share with her husband.

Men such as John often attribute real health problems to aging. It's important to determine if there is a deteriorating quality of life issue. So Dr. Lamm asks him key questions about his daily health now as compared to 10 or 20 years ago. What is his energy level? Does he exercise and, if so, how much can he tolerate? Are his interest in sex and level of sexual performance the same?

But perhaps the single best question to put to John is this: "Are you having regular morning erections?" As doctors, that is a sign to us that a man's heart and blood vessels, nervous system, hormones, and sleep patterns are all likely working well. If a man says no, it's a red flag that something probably isn't as it should be.

When John reports that he hasn't had a morning erection in months, it's time to start digging a bit deeper. Let's look at the role of the prostate in the male body, common prostate problems that may be troubling John, and the lifestyle changes we can recommend to be sure that John is doing all he can to protect against prostate cancer and live a healthy and fulfilling life.

A Prostate Primer

The prostate is a smooth, firm gland located just under the bladder and in front of the rectum. It surrounds a portion of the urethra, the tube that passes urine from the bladder through the penis and out of the body. Small ducts, or tiny tube-like openings, pass from the prostate into the urethra (see figure 1).

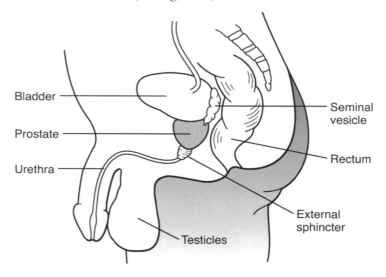

Figure 1. Anatomy of the prostate.

The prostate is there primarily for reproductive reasons. It works with the seminal vesicles, two small glands that sit behind and just above it, to produce semen—the fluid that carries sperm. This fluid makes it easier to propel sperm through the vagina and uterus and also serves to protect the sperm from the acidic environment of the vagina. During male orgasm, muscles in the prostate push this fluid out into the urethra, where it mixes with other semen components and sperm and leaves the body during ejaculation.

Size Matters

Men are born with a pea-sized prostate. During puberty, the prostate has a short growth spurt. By early adulthood, the prostate is about the size of a walnut. But around age 25, the prostate starts to grow again, making it the only gland that almost always increases in size as we age. We aren't completely sure why this happens; one popular theory is that it is due to shifts in hormone balance as men age.

It's important to note that this growth is normal and is not by itself a sign of illness or cancer. You may not be aware of prostate enlargement for many years. Or, you may notice minor lower urinary tract symptoms (LUTS) that, while irksome, don't really affect your quality of life.

But in some cases, a growing or enlarged prostate can cause health problems, making it impossible to ignore for many men. The prostate can push into the bladder and/or urethra, interfering with urine flow (see figure 2). As a result, a man may strain to urinate and have problems completely emptying his bladder. His sleep quality may be disrupted due to frequent awakening to urinate. His urine flow may be sporadic. In some cases, incontinence (urine leakage or dribbling) can also result. This condition is known as benign prostatic hyperplasia (BPH).

Common Prostate Problems

Most prostate problems are not cancer related. Statistically, men are more likely to experience BPH or prostatitis (swelling and inflammation) than a serious prostate cancer. Let's look at the most common prostate conditions in men and how to recognize them.

Benign Prostatic Hyperplasia

BPH is the most common prostate health problem in men over 50 years of age. It is characterized by a group of urinary problems called lower urinary tract symptoms (LUTS). According to the National Institutes of Health, BPH affects about half of men over age 50 and up to 90% of men age 70 and older.

Symptoms of BPH may include:
- a weak or erratic urine flow
- trouble starting and stopping urination
- frequent urination that may interrupt normal activity and sleep
- small amounts of urine when you do go to the bathroom
- a feeling like you still need to urinate, even though you just did
- dribbling or leaking urine
- frequent urinary tract infections
- acute or chronic urinary retention

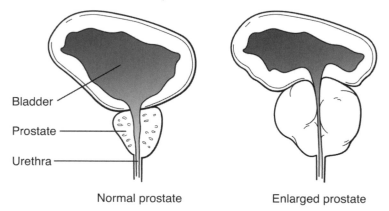

Bladder

Prostate

Urethra

Normal prostate   Enlarged prostate

Figure 2. Comparison of a normal and enlarged prostate.

The symptoms of BPH may be treated with medication designed to improve urinary flow. Other drugs decrease the size of the prostate and stop further growth. For some men with severe BPH that doesn't respond to drug treatment, surgery is an option. There are several methods of surgery, but all involve removal of the prostate tissue that is blocking the urethra. There are also other minimally invasive methods of destroying the troublesome prostate tissue with heat to restore normal urine flow through the urethra.

Prostatitis

Prostatitis (irritation or inflammation/swelling) is the most common prostate issue in men under 50 years of age. Like BPH, it causes quite a few problems with urination. But unlike BPH, it is also usually accompanied by pain, which may be in the groin, genitals, abdomen, or lower back.

In most cases we don't know what triggers the inflammatory process. It may be an immune system reaction. Prostatitis may be caused by a bacterial infection. Bacterial prostatitis can usually be effectively treated with a course of antibiotics, either short or long. A combination of muscle relaxing drugs, pain relievers, and massage techniques may be recommended to reduce non-bacterial prostatitis discomfort.

Symptoms of prostatitis include:
- a weak or erratic urine flow
- pain or burning during urination
- trouble starting and stopping urination
- frequent urination that may interrupt normal activity and sleep
- small amounts of urine when you do go to the bathroom
- a feeling like you still need to urinate, even though you just did
- dribbling or leaking urine
- pain in the abdomen, groin, genitals, or lower back
- painful orgasms
- flu symptoms such as fever and aches (with bacterial prostatitis only)

Prostate Cancer

And then there is prostate cancer, which is probably the reason you've picked up this book. It is the second most common cause of cancer death in men, but also the most highly treatable. Most prostate cancers are found in early stages in men age 65 and older. The five-year survival rate for men diagnosed with early-stage localized (i.e., confined to the prostate) prostate cancer is 100%.[1] The odds don't get much better than that.

Early-stage prostate cancer rarely causes any symptoms. If symptoms do exist, it may be because of preexisting BPH. So screening to catch it early, when the cancer is "curable," is important.

The trouble with prostate cancer is that there is not yet a really good screening test for it. The best to which we currently have access—the prostate-specific antigen (PSA) test—is not very sensitive or specific. When we use the PSA test, we do find potentially lethal prostate cancers, but we also end up with an unacceptable number of false positives and false negatives. That is, we end up suspecting prostate cancer in men who don't have it, and we miss prostate cancers in men who do have it. That is why PSA screening is not right for everyone (a topic we'll discuss in detail in chapter 2). The bottom line for doctors and patients is that it's important to administer this test in an intelligent way, taking into account each man's individual lifestyle and health history and using advanced imaging tools when appropriate.

Prostate Changes and Age

It may sound as if the prostate pretty much takes care of itself and will let you know if there's a problem by having your life revolve around urgently finding a bathroom. However, most men with early-stage prostate cancer have no symptoms, and prostate cancer is typically very slow growing compared to other cancers. It can take decades before a tumor grows large enough to be felt with a rectal exam or cause any noticeable problems.

Add to this the fact that men aren't particularly proactive about their health care and you see the dilemma. When older men experience changes in prostate health, such as more frequent urination and weak urine flow, they often attribute it to age and assume there's nothing to be done but learn to live with it. Yet these same issues can be a sign of a serious health problem, including advanced prostate cancer.

So how do we catch prostate changes early enough to treat them, without causing men undue stress and unnecessary procedures?

Changing the Male Perspective on Healthcare

Let's return to our patient John. He's seeing the doctor at his wife's request and is not particularly concerned about any health problems. He feels fine "for his age," and while he knows he has a few pounds to lose, he expects everything to check out fine. From his perspective, he probably won't need to return to the doctor for another 15 years. This is another thing to check off his "to do" list.

Until he is asked about his morning erections. He struggles to remember the last time he had one. Perhaps a month ago? Maybe two? Come to think of it, sex was a bit more of a chore lately. He didn't realize that, at 58, morning erections should be a regular occurrence. He wonders if his wife has noticed any difference? And suddenly, we have his attention.

Statistically, men are less likely to seek a doctor's care for health problems, to "soldier on" past health disruptions even when it's clearly not in their best interest to do so.[2] This can often mean that we don't seek help for a problem early enough to effectively treat it. But most men under the age of 75 do sit up and take notice when their sexual health is at stake.[3]

It's not just the psychological makeup of men that creates this gender bias against preventive healthcare. It's also the way our healthcare system is set up. As children, most American girls and boys see a pediatrician regularly until around age 18. Then young women typically transition to an obstetrician/gynecologist for continuing regular care.

But men often drop out of the system, seeking care only when faced with acute illness or injury, until they reach an age when health issues force them back into the system ... or a concerned spouse or significant other does. John is not unusual in this respect.

As physicians, we recognize that a renewed focus on men's health throughout the life span is extremely important. Many doctors and hospitals are establishing programs to close this men's healthcare gap. For example, one of your authors, Dr. Lamm, is the Director of Men's Health at New York University Medical Center, a large urban medical facility that is trying to encourage a more engaged male patient.

Once John recognizes and shares his issues, we can take a course of action. We check his testosterone levels, the male reproductive hormone that is closely tied to prostate health, and assess his cardiovascular health with blood pressure and cholesterol tests. And we decide that, given John's age and lifestyle, it makes sense to order a prostate-specific antigen (PSA) test to check for prostate cancer.

With John, it was important to reset his expectations about aging and settling for a less fulfilling life. Aging should not be about what you "can't do." Your quality of life, energy level, and sexual performance should stay high. And there are often simple ways to fix problems early on.

Prostate Maintenance

All of the things you know you should do to protect your health—regular exercise, quitting smoking, maintaining a healthy weight and waist circumference (40 inches or less), and eating a balanced and healthy diet—are good for your prostate, as well. There is substantial research on prostate cancer prevention and lifestyle health, and many excellent books are devoted to the subject. Following are a few pointers on how eating, moving, and maintaining your mental balance can promote prostate health. Talk to your healthcare provider about how to fit these into your lifestyle.

Nutrition

All fruits and vegetables have health benefits, and many have anti-inflammatory or anti-oxidative properties that are protective against cancer. Eat a variety of both in their fresh, unprocessed form whenever possible.

Despite the known anti-inflammatory properties of omega-3 fatty acids, there has been a recent report on the association of omega-3s and prostate cancer. It is important to note that association does not mean causality. Speak to your physician on the risk-benefit ratio of omega-3 fatty acids.

Limit animal fats in your diet and, when you do eat meat or poultry, take care not to overcook it. Grilled and well-done meat may contain carcinogens that promote prostate cancer.[4]

Finally, cut your intake of sugar and other highly processed carbohydrates. They promote weight and fat gain and feed tumor growth.[5]

Are there any foods that may protect against prostate cancer?

Foods rich in antioxidants and other phytochemicals are thought to be protective against many cancers. These include fruits and vegetables across the color spectrum, from ruby-red lycopene-rich tomatoes to deep green veggies that contain compounds that help the liver break down carcinogens. Other all-star foods include green tea, pomegranates, and soy.

Exercise

How can exercise help your prostate health? It fights the inflammatory and oxidative processes that fuel cancer. Muscle mass tends to diminish as we age, which can affect our overall health, so weight training and regular movement that strengthen our bodies are important for this reason, as well. Finally, exercising helps improve our mental functioning and can relieve stress—a known culprit in diminishing overall health and accelerating existing cancer growth.

Aim for one hour of exercise daily. This can be anything from long walks to scheduled gym visits to participating in team sports. Do what you enjoy and you'll be more likely to keep up with it.

Stress Reduction

Stress is a part of all of our lives. But learning how to effectively handle it can make a dramatic difference in our health and happiness. Stress triggers a chemical response within the body that weakens our immune systems.[6] And studies have shown that these stress chemicals can inhibit the ability of some cancer drugs to kill prostate cancer cells.

I've heard that stress can cause prostate cancer. Is that true?

Stress cannot be blamed as a direct cause for prostate cancer. However, there is a substantial body of evidence that ties chronic stress to a long list of health problems, from anxiety disorders to heart disease. In addition, the physical effects of stress have been shown to accelerate prostate cancer tumor growth in animal studies.[7]

Putting It All Together

In John's case, his laboratory tests and physical exam reveal that he is 20 pounds overweight, has borderline high blood pressure, high total cholesterol, and low HDL (good) cholesterol. His PSA is 1 ng/mL, which is considered normal, but his testosterone levels are low.

Testosterone levels do tend to drop as we age, but the good news is that with supplementation (a daily prescription dose of the hormone), we can bring John's levels back into a normal range. We will keep an eye on his PSA levels over time, as an increase in testosterone levels typically causes a rise in PSA and could be a marker for prostate cancer problems.

We also make lifestyle recommendations for John to improve his cholesterol levels and blood pressure—diet, exercise, and stress reduction. It's interesting to note that these are the same changes that keep your prostate healthy and, in some cases, protect against prostate cancer. John returns to the office six months later, experiencing the benefits of following the lifestyle changes—increased energy and improved sexual performance. He reports feeling "20 years younger," has lost 15 pounds, and says his wife is thrilled with the changes she sees in him. We applaud his success, but also encourage him to keep up with his healthy lifestyle habits, as at least 80% of people regain the weight they lose. Health maintenance is, indeed, a daily, lifelong task.

References

1. Howlader N, Noone AM, Krapcho M, et al. (eds).
   SEER Cancer Statistics Review, 1975-2009 (Vintage 2009 Populations),
   National Cancer Institute. Bethesda, MD,
   http://seer.cancer.gov/csr/1975_2009_pops09/, based on November
   2011 SEER data submission, posted to the SEER web site, 2012.
2. Pinkhasov RM, Wong J, Kashanian J, et al. Are men shortchanged
   on health? Perspective on health care utilization and health risk
   behavior in men and women in the United States. *Int J Clin Pract.*
   2010 Mar;64(4):475–87.
   doi: 10.1111/j.1742-1241.2009.02290.x. Review.
3. Tannenbaum C. Effect of age, education and health status on
   community dwelling older men's health concerns. *Aging Male.*
   2012 Jun;15(2):103–8.
4. Cross AJ, Peters U, Kirsh VA, et al. A prospective study of meat
   and meat mutagens and prostate cancer risk. *Cancer Res.*
   2005;65:11779–11784.
5. Freedland SJ, Mavrooulos J, Wang A, et al. Carbohydrate restriction,
   prostate cancer growth, and the insulin-like growth factor axis.
   Prostate. 2008;68:11–19.
6. Nagaraja AS, Armaiz-Pena GN, Lutgendorf SK, Sood AK.
   Why stress is BAD for cancer patients. *J Clin Invest.* 2013 Jan; 25:1–3.
7. Hassan S, Karpova Y, Baiz D, et al. Behavioral stress accelerates
   prostate cancer development in mice. *J Clin Invest.*
   2013 Feb 1;123(2):874-86. doi: 10.1172/JCI63324. Epub 2013 Jan 25.

Patient Checklist

Bring this checklist with you to your next doctor's visit to get the answers you need to stay healthy. See the chapter 2 "Patient Checklist" for questions to ask about PSA testing.

☐ Is my prostate enlarged? Does this pose a health risk for me at this point in time? _____

_____

☐ How can I treat urinary problems at home? _____

_____

☐ Do I need medication for prostate problems? What are the risks and benefits? _____

_____

☐ Do my prostate problems increase my risk of prostate cancer? _____

_____

☐ Given my health and family history, age, and lifestyle, what is my individual risk for prostate cancer? _____

_____

☐ Should I be making any dietary or lifestyle changes to keep my prostate healthy? _____

_____

☐ When should I return for a follow-up visit? How often should I be getting my prostate checked? _____

_____

_____

Visit www.sprypubprostate.com to download a printable checklist.

CHAPTER TWO

Checking Your Prostate: What's Right for You?

One Man's Story

Frank is a 52-year-old man with a wife and two children ages 17 and 15. He feels healthy, enjoys his job, and is living a full and happy life. As an engineer, Frank is well read and fairly inquisitive. Recently, he read an article about prostate cancer screening with the PSA blood test and new recommendations against "routine" screening. When he goes in for his annual physical, he questions his doctor about the need for a PSA test.

From what Frank has read, there are experts on both sides of the issue. Some claim that studies fail to show any benefit of PSA screening and that the blood test doesn't save lives. In addition, a PSA level can be high for many reasons unrelated to cancer, and that leads to unnecessary biopsies and invasive treatment for many men, which can have serious side effects. On the other side of the fence, advocates of the test point to an almost 40% decline in prostate cancer mortality since PSA screening became available.[1]

When Frank asked about the PSA controversy, his doctor seemed conflicted. He acknowledged that there were contradictory opinions on the pros and cons of PSA screening. The office was busy, as usual, which also limited his discussion with Frank. He gave a quick answer: "I had my PSA checked. I suggest you do, as well." So, Frank made a quick decision and had his blood drawn, even though he was still uncertain if he was doing the right thing.

One week later, Frank received a call from his doctor. The laboratory results showed that his PSA was 6.2 ng/mL. His doctor advised him that while this elevated level was important to follow up on, the PSA test is not perfect and the elevation could be caused by a number of things. Frank was referred to a urologist to discuss the next steps.

Why Screen for Prostate Cancer?

Why do we screen for any cancer? In their earliest stages, most cancers start out as a small lesion confined to one part of the body (e.g., prostate, breast, bladder, lung). It is at this early stage that potentially lethal cancers should be found and treated in order to be reliably cured. Treatment involves either surgically removing the cancerous tissue or destroying it using radiation, heat, or other methods. Because most cancers do not produce any physical signs or cause symptoms when they are small, we rely on screening tests to find and treat them.

If left untreated, over time most cancers will metastasize (or spread) to other parts of the body and ultimately cause death. These metastases invade other vital organs, and symptoms such as weight loss, pain, and fatigue develop. The spread of some cancers can be stopped using potent chemotherapy. Unfortunately, in most cases, chemotherapy only halts the disease temporarily.

A chairman of gynecology at a major medical institution once said that prostate cancer is "a great cancer to live with, but a terrible cancer to die with." We spend our lives counseling men on their health, and this is the primary reason why we feel prostate cancer screening is so very critical to catch cancer in its earliest, treatable stages. For some of us, it has a more personal connotation; Dr. Lamm watched his father, also a physician, suffer with and eventually pass away from late-stage metastasized prostate cancer. Dr. Lepor observed a similar scenario with his uncle.

In general, screening is reserved for those cancers that are common in the general population, highly treatable, and associated with high mortality rates—such as lung, colon, and breast cancer. Prostate cancer fits all of these criteria. It is the second most common cause of cancer mortality among American males. In 2013, it is estimated that 29,720 American men will lose their lives to prostate cancer.[2] Again, because it causes no symptoms and cannot be easily detected on physical examination in its early stages when it is most treatable, appropriate screening for prostate cancer is very important.

However, it's important to understand that not every prostate cancer is lethal. Unlike more aggressive cancers (e.g., lung, pancreatic), prostate cancer is typically slow growing and in some cases may not pose a threat to health or life. A common turn of phrase in the field of men's health is that "more men die *with* prostate cancer than *from* prostate cancer." If detected early, there is a wide window of time in which to treat it. So again, having access to prostate cancer screening is important.

To be effective, a screening test should:

- **Be Accessible**—Low cost and ease of use ensure that a screening test is widely available to the general population.
- **Have High Sensitivity**—The test should able to identify the majority of people who have a cancer that will become lethal and not miss an existing cancer (known as a false-negative result).
- **Have High Specificity**—The test should zero in on only those affected by the cancer and not incorrectly identify those who are cancer free as having cancer (known as a false-positive result).

The Digital Rectal Examination

The Test No One Wants, But Men Over 40 Need

The digital rectal examination (DRE) is a simple test with which most older men are already familiar. It is performed by the doctor inserting a finger into the rectum and palpating (feeling) the prostate gland (see figure 3). Cancers on DRE will feel hard in comparison to the smooth, rubbery tissue of a normal prostate gland. All men over the age of 40 years old should undergo a DRE as part of a physical examination.

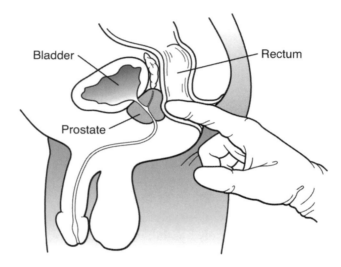

Figure 3. Digital rectal examination.
The normal prostate gland should feel smooth and rubbery.

However, the DRE allows your doctor to examine only one portion of the prostate gland (the part that is located next to the rectum), so any tumors in other parts of the prostate will be missed by a DRE. In addition, most early prostate cancers usually can't be felt on DRE. Finally, the usefulness of this test is very dependent on a doctor's skill and experience. For these reasons, DRE alone is not an adequate strategy for screening for early prostate cancer.

My PSA is normal ... do I need a digital rectal examination?

A digital rectal exam is an important part of a comprehensive prostate cancer screening strategy, regardless of PSA results. One study of more than 800 men found that 31% had an abnormal DRE and normal PSA.[3] One well-known example is that of the late General Norman Schwarzkopf. In 1996, his urologist found a small nodule on his prostate during a routine DRE. General Schwarzkopf had just had a PSA test with normal results, but after the DRE he underwent an ultrasound and prostate biopsy at his urologist's suggestion to be safe. The diagnosis was prostate cancer.[4] After successful radical prostatectomy treatment, the general was cancer free when he passed away from complications of pneumonia in 2012 at the age of 78.

What Is PSA?

Prostate-specific antigen (PSA) is a protein that is produced by the prostate. The name has turned out to be somewhat of a misnomer, as in the past few decades researchers have discovered that women also produce trace levels of PSA in breast tissue.[5]

In men, PSA is a component of ejaculate and is found in small amounts in the blood of healthy men. When the prostate is diseased or damaged, levels of PSA in the bloodstream may rise.

Very low levels of PSA can be detected in the blood using inexpensive laboratory tests, which makes PSA screening a useful and noninvasive test for spotting early signs of trouble in the prostate. The primary limitation of PSA as a screening tool for prostate cancer is that it lacks specificity. In other words, a high PSA level could mean prostate cancer, but it could also be a sign of enlargement, infection, inflammation, or injury to the prostate unrelated to cancer. Common conditions of the prostate that can increase PSA levels include benign prostatic hyperplasia and prostatitis.

The problem with this, and one of the reasons the U.S. Preventive

Services Task Force (USPSTF) currently recommends against routine PSA screening for prostate cancer, is that many men with benign (non-cancerous) conditions of the prostate end up undergoing unnecessary and invasive diagnostic testing for cancer. These unnecessary tests pose a health risk to the patient, can have unpleasant side effects, cause anxiety, and are expensive. In addition, the detection of non-lethal cancers may lead to unnecessary treatment.

What is considered a "normal" level of PSA?

What is considered normal will vary by age, ethnicity, and health history of each man. Results may also vary by laboratory assay (test) used. So there are no global "normal" values that apply to all men. But to give you some general idea, the following table lists age-specific reference ranges published by the American Urological Association:

Serum PSA Reference Ranges

Age Range	Asian-Americans	African-Americans	Caucasian
40–49	≤2.0 ng/mL	≤2.0 ng/mL	≤2.5 ng/mL
50–59	≤3.0 ng/mL	≤4.0 ng/mL	≤3.5 ng/mL
60–69	≤4.0 ng/mL	≤4.5 ng/mL	≤4.5 ng/mL
70–79	≤5.0 ng/mL	≤5.5 ng/mL	≤6.5 ng/mL

Source: American Urological Association;
Prostate-specific antigen best practice statement.[6]

But again, the PSA value by itself is not enough information to determine whether a prostate biopsy is needed, since a high PSA can be a sign of a non-cancerous condition. The PSA density (PSAD), free PSA, and the PSA velocity (PSAV) are values to know in under-standing your prostate cancer risk.

PSA Density and Free PSA

In general, men with larger prostate glands have higher PSA levels. Because we know not every large prostate is cancerous, we try to adjust for this with a calculation known as the PSA density (PSAD). The PSAD is determined by first establishing the prostate volume (size) with an ultrasound scan, and then dividing the PSA level by this volume. The higher the PSAD, the higher the cancer risk.

Another important PSA parameter is "free PSA." PSA may exist bound to proteins or free in the blood serum. A lower percentage of free PSA is associated with a greater chance that a high PSA level is associated with cancer. Interpretation of the free PSA depends on the type of laboratory assay used.

PSA Velocity

PSA velocity (PSAV) is the rate at which the PSA increases from one PSA test to the next. Velocity may provide important insights into interpreting PSA levels, although some doctors disagree on the usefulness of this measurement. Since the prostate grows very slowly, a high PSA caused by BPH should increase very slowly over time. For a condition like prostatitis, the inflammation of the prostate would cause wide swings in the PSA level.

Those prostate cancers that are clinically significant grow steadily. The specific rate of change (PSA velocity) that could indicate prostate cancer is about 0.5 ng/mL/year. For example, a PSA history over three years of 2.0, 2.6, 3.2 ng/mL has a strong possibility of being prostate cancer. On the other hand, annual PSA levels of 4.0, 3.8, 4.1 ng/mL would be consistent with non-cancerous changes. It's important to realize that different guidelines for these values exist; the American Urological Association (AUA) uses a marker of greater than 0.4 ng/mL/year and the National Comprehensive Cancer Network (NCCN) says greater than 0.35 ng/mL/year.[7,8]

My PSA came back high. Should I get my PSA retested before I agree to a biopsy?

Every test is subject to possible laboratory error. If your first PSA is elevated then it should be repeated to confirm the test is abnormal. If there is a history of normal PSAs and a subsequent test is markedly higher, again the test should be repeated to confirm the change in PSA. For accurate results, men should not ejaculate 72 hours prior to having a PSA test.

Remember that many things can raise your PSA level besides prostate cancer. These include:

- **Urinary Tract Infection (UTI)**—Your doctor should be able to diagnose a UTI with a simple urine test.
- **Benign Prostatic Hyperplasia or Enlargement**—The larger the prostate, the greater chance PSA elevation may be due to a benign and not malignant condition.
- **Prostatitis**—Inflammation of the prostate can cause a rise in PSA.

The PSA Controversy: Pros and Cons

The USPSTF is a federally appointed, independent committee of healthcare professionals whose responsibility is to make recommendations on guidelines for clinical preventive services, including cancer screening. When task force members reissued prostate cancer screening guidelines in 2012, they based them on the available clinical research. The USPSTF recommended against routine prostate screening for all men, concluding that the risk of unnecessary procedures outweighed the benefits of early cancer detection.[9]

It's important to note that USPSTF members do not specialize in prostate cancer, and there were no urologists, medical oncologists, or radiation oncologists on the task force that authored these recommendations. However, the USPSTF does invite these specialists and others to submit comments for consideration before final guidelines are issued.

Since the USPSTF screening recommendation was made, the American College of Physicians (ACP) has issued revised guidelines against routine PSA screening.[10] But other professional clinical organizations, including the American Medical Association, have publicly voiced their opposition to the USPSTF conclusions. Unfortunately, this has resulted in a lot of confusion for you, the patient. Why the lack of agreement? Let's take a look at the research behind PSA screening.

The Research

One of the major studies the USPSTF considered in their recommendations was the Prostate, Lung, Colorectal, and Ovarian (PLCO) Cancer Screening Trial. The PLCO was an attempt to determine whether regular screening for prostate, lung, colorectal, and ovarian cancers resulted in a lower death rate among people with these diseases.[11]

More than 76,000 men at ten U.S. centers were enrolled in this study between 1993 and 2001. The study participants were put into one of the two groups at random. Half of the men were assigned to a routine of annual PSA prostate cancer screening and half were assigned to a control group without prescribed screening.

Those men assigned to the PSA screening arm were advised to undergo PSA testing annually for six years and annual DRE for four years. Those in the control group were advised not to undergo regular screening. There were no standard protocols for when to perform a biopsy for an "abnormal" PSA and how to treat those men diagnosed with prostate cancer.

While a greater number of men were diagnosed with prostate cancer in the PSA group, there was no significant difference in overall mortality or prostate cancer mortality in the group that received regular screening. The study results, reported in the *New England Journal of Medicine*, therefore concluded that annual PSA screening does not save lives.[12]

So, if the PLCO study failed to show a benefit for PSA screening why is there a controversy? Simply put, the PLCO study was flawed as a true analysis of the usefulness of PSA screening for a number of reasons.

1. The PLCO had a high degree of study contamination. This means that men were exposed to the intervention being evaluated (in this case, PSA screening) when they should not have been for a truly unbiased, well-powered clinical trial. Specifically, 44% of all men enrolled in the trial had already undergone PSA screening prior to the study, so many had benefitted from PSA screening before the trial even began. And more than 80% of men randomized to the control arm underwent PSA testing.

2. Half of the men with an elevated PSA did not undergo prostate biopsy.[13]

3. Many men diagnosed with prostate cancer during the study chose not to undergo treatment.

4. The study term of 7–10 years follow-up is inadequate to ascertain the survival benefit of early detection by PSA screening. Although the PLCO trial has planned a future follow-up of all study subjects at 13 years, prostate cancer is slow growing and a study term of at least 15 years would be required to accurately determine long-term survival benefits. Ideally, men who are in their 40s at diagnosis would require a 40-year study since this is the time they would be at risk from their disease.

5. Preventing development of life-threatening metastasis is a key benefit of early prostate cancer detection, and the PLCO trial did not evaluate how this affected the overall death rate.

The European Randomized Study of Screening for Prostate Cancer (ERSPC) enrolled 184,000 men in eight countries into a study examining whether PSA screening prevents prostate cancer mortality. The European trial also randomized men to either a PSA screening group or a control (non-screening) group.

From a trial design standpoint, the ERSPC is stronger and has far less contamination than the PLCO study. In the ERSPC, fewer men had undergone screening prior to enrollment, fewer control subjects underwent PSA screening, and the follow-up was longer. The ERSPC found that PSA screening resulted in a 29% reduction in prostate cancer mortality.[14]

The Göteborg Randomised Population-Based Prostate-Cancer Screening Trial, which later became a subset of the ERSPC trial, was a study of 20,000 Swedish men age 50–64 to assess the effects of PSA prostate cancer screening every two years. This trial, which ran from 1994 to 2008, provides the greatest insights into the benefits of PSA screening, since screening had not been widely adopted in Sweden at the start of the trial. This meant that very few men underwent PSA screening prior to enrollment, and very few control subjects underwent screening (so study contamination was extremely low). The Göteborg trial found that PSA screening reduced prostate cancer mortality by about half at 14-year follow-up.[15]

Perhaps the best evidence for the value of PSA screening in reducing death rates from prostate cancer can be found by looking at the history of screening here in the United States. PSA was first identified as a prostate cancer marker in the late 1970s. The first studies showing the benefits of PSA screening for the purpose of early prostate cancer detection were published in the early 1990s.[16] In 1994, the U.S. Food and Drug Administration (FDA) approved the first PSA test for early prostate cancer detection, and testing became widely adopted by physicians shortly thereafter.

Knowing what we do about how prostate cancer grows, any survival benefits of PSA screening would not begin to appear until about a decade after widespread adoption of the PSA test. This is exactly what has been observed in the U.S. population. Widespread prostate cancer screening became available in the 1990s, and between 1992 and 2007, the prostate cancer mortality rate decreased by 40%.[17] There is no other factor that can explain the decrease in prostate cancer mortality other than adoption of PSA screening. The observations in the U.S. population also correspond with the findings of the Göteborg trial. Simply put, prostate cancer screening saves lives.

Should I Get a PSA Test?

So, what do we do today as far as screening? Abandoning PSA testing would take us back to the time when prostate cancer was a death sentence and is clearly not an option. What does make sense is to use the tools we have in more intelligent ways; to screen and detect smarter and to educate and involve you, the patient, on the implications of PSA and other screening methods to your life.

The age to begin testing is controversial even among those who recommend PSA screening. Some recommend beginning annual PSA screening for men without risk factors at age 50. Others recommend annual PSA screening for all men beginning at age 40.

An interesting new study out of Memorial Sloan-Kettering Cancer Center of over 21,000 Swedish men found that, by measuring PSA levels at age 45, most men who are at long-term risk of aggressive cancers can be identified for regular continued screening. For the rest (roughly half of all men), having just three PSA tests—in a man's 40s, early 50s, and finally at age 60—is sufficient.[18] If further research bears out these findings, it could be a big step forward in reducing the rate of over-diagnosis and over-treatment of prostate cancer in men.

As this book went to press, the American Urological Association (AUA) issued new guidelines for prostate cancer screening that focus on shared decision making between doctors and patients. The AUA recommends that men age 55 to 69 who are considering prostate cancer screening talk with their doctors about the benefits and harms of routine testing in light of their personal values and preferences. For those men who choose screening, the AUA recommends a screening interval of every two years versus annually. The AUA also recommends against PSA screening in men under age 40 and against routine screening in average-risk men between the ages of 40 and 54. It also advises against routine screening in men over age 70 or with a life expectancy of less than 10 to 15 years.[19]

The failure to recommend screening for men between the ages of 40 to 54 is not based on evidence failing to show benefit, but rather a lack of clinical evidence in this cohort of men. Despite the lack of evidence, many believe that men between 40 and 54 are the ideal group for PSA screening since there is less PSA produced by BPH, and slow-growing cancers likely pose a risk for these men with long life expectancies.

So what's the bottom line? Based on the clinical evidence and our own experience with a combined 60+ years of practice, we feel the evidence supports annual PSA screening for men who:

- are age 40 or older and considered at high risk (i.e., a family history of prostate cancer, African-American)
- have a life expectancy of more than 10 years.

For men who are not high risk, if the PSA is normal then screening may be performed every 2 years.

Based upon current life expectancy tables, the average life expectancy of a 70-year-old American man is 14.3 years.[20] When considering a patient's life expectancy, we look at their family history and full health picture. A 75-year-old man with no major health problems whose parents are still alive may benefit from a PSA test, while it's possible a younger 70-year-old man with heart disease, uncontrolled diabetes, and no living relatives may not.

The Future of PSA Screening

The major issue with prostate cancer screening today is that, following an elevated PSA test, too many men who do not have prostate cancer are being subjected to a biopsy. We obviously need a better screening tool than PSA, one that is specific to potentially lethal prostate cancers. Unfortunately, it may be some time before that happens. In the meantime, free PSA, PSAD, and PSA velocity can be used strategically to hone in on a man's cancer risk. And, of course, it's important for doctors to consider their individual patient; to look at a man's age, lifestyle, and health history to help him make more informed decisions about whether or not to get a biopsy.

Another problem with our prostate cancer detection strategy is the random tissue sampling biopsy that is currently the standard of care for prostate cancer diagnosis in the United States. This technique, which is discussed in detail in chapter 4, can miss lethal cancers in those parts of the prostate that are not sampled. It can also detect cancers that are of no real threat. But in the case of biopsy, unlike screening, we do have tools at our disposal that can avoid these issues. Advanced imaging techniques such as multiparametric magnetic resonance imaging (mpMRI) can detect and target cancerous areas with greater accuracy. The Smilow Comprehensive Prostate Cancer Center at NYU Langone Medical Center, under the direction of Dr. Lepor, is one of the leading centers investigating this promising adjunct to PSA screening.

In 2012, the U.S. Food and Drug Administration (FDA) gave premarket approval for a new test called the Prostate Health Index (*phi*). It is not meant to replace the PSA, but rather to supplement it for men 50 years and older who have PSA results of 4–10 ng/mL and a negative digital rectal exam. The *phi* measures components of PSA, including total PSA and free PSA. It also measures a subcategory of free PSA called pro-PSA (or p2PSA), which is thought to be closely tied to prostate cancer. The *phi* is designed to help distinguish whether an elevated PSA level is due to cancer or benign conditions such as prostatitis and BPH. The test manufacturer, Beckman Coulter, reports that in multicenter clinical trials the *phi* test reduced unnecessary biopsies by 31%.[21] More large controlled studies are needed to determine the effectiveness of this test in identifying prostate cancer.

Gene-Based Testing

The Prostate Cancer Antigen 3 Gene

The prostate cancer antigen 3 (PCA3) test is a simple urine test that detects a genetic material released by prostate cancer cells. It is performed immediately following a DRE. The higher a PCA3 score, the more likely a follow-up prostate biopsy will be positive for cancer.

The PCA3 is *not* a replacement for PSA testing, but is an additional tool to use to guide your treatment decisions.

When a patient has a high PSA, the PCA3 can be useful in further zeroing in on their prostate cancer risk. If the PCA3 results are also high, that is another indication that cancer may be present and biopsy may be appropriate. If the PCA3 is low, then it's possible that a non-cancerous prostate condition is causing the rise in PSA, and biopsy may not be necessary.

Some studies have indicated that the PCA3 may also be helpful in detecting not just the presence of prostate cancer, but also how aggressive the cancer may be. To date, the test is only FDA approved for determining who should undergo a second prostate cancer biopsy when the first biopsy is negative.

Should I have a PCA3 test before my biopsy?

Dr. Lepor answers: "In my practice, it is standard to run a PCA3 test on all men with an elevated PSA before biopsy. I also order a multiparametric MRI, or mpMRI, to get a better look at the prostate. If the PCA3 and mpMRI are negative, then in selected cases I will not recommend a biopsy. But if the PSA velocity is increasing steadily or there is a family history of prostate cancer in this group, I will usually go ahead with a biopsy despite a negative PCA3 and mpMRI. I will then use the mpMRI to guide my biopsy." mpMRI imaging and biopsy are described in detail in chapter 4 of this book.

Other Genetic Tests

The Oncotype DX (Genomic Health) is a test that is performed on the biopsy tissue sample. It uses an algorithm to generate a score known as the genomic prostate score (GPS), which predicts the likelihood that a patient's early-stage prostate cancer will grow and spread. While it may have clinical utility for some men, this test can be costly and is not always covered by insurance. Its accuracy is also limited by the sampling error of the biopsy sample itself.

Another genetic biomarker known as TMPRSS2:ERG (developed by Hologic Gen-Probe) has shown promising results for the risk stratification of men with high PSA values when used in combination with PCA3 testing. In early trials, this simple urine test was found to predict the presence of higher-risk cancers with similar accuracy to biopsy outcome.[22] This test is still in the research phase and has not yet been submitted to the U.S. FDA for approval.

There is no doubt we will ultimately have better screening tools for prostate cancer. In the meantime, the challenge is to use the tools we do have to our best advantage. Figure 4 illustrates the current testing and thought processes that lead from the first PSA test/DRE to a potential biopsy.

Putting It All Together

Frank is referred to a urologist, Dr. Lepor, who repeats the PSA test, which remains elevated. He recommends a PCA3 test and an mpMRI imaging scan of the prostate. The PCA3 is elevated and the mpMRI shows a highly suspicious area in the right lobe of the prostate.

The urologist tells Frank that these results indicate a strong possibility of prostate cancer and recommends biopsy of the suspicious area. Using a novel biopsy technique that combines mpMRI with a three-dimensional ultrasound image (described in detail in chapter 4), the urologist is able to accurately target the suspicious area for biopsy.

After biopsy, a Gleason 7 cancer was diagnosed. The urologist discusses all treatment options with Frank, who decides on surgery to remove his prostate gland (a radical prostatectomy). He had temporary but expected side effects of incontinence and erectile dysfunction. Two years later, these complications have resolved and his PSA level is currently undetectable. In Frank's case, PSA screening was a lifesaver.

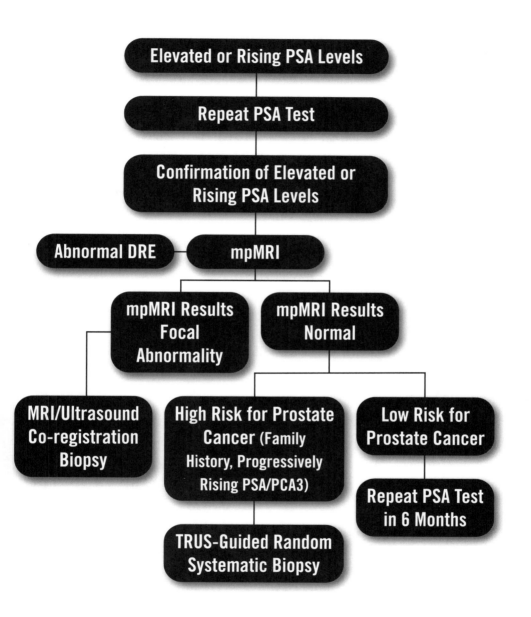

Figure 4. Decision tree for prostate biopsy.

References

1. Stephenson RA. Prostate cancer trends in the era of prostate-specific antigen. An update of incidence, mortality, and clinical factors from the SEER database. *Urol Clin North Am.* 2002 Feb;29(1):173–81.

2. Siegel R, Naishadham D, Jemal A. Cancer statistics, 2013. *CA: A Cancer Journal for Clinicians.* 63:11–30. doi: 10.3322/caac.21166.

3. Palmerola R, Smith P, Elliot V, et al. The digital rectal examination (DRE) remains important—outcomes from a contemporary cohort of men undergoing an initial 12-18 core prostate needle biopsy. *Can J Urol.* 2012 Dec;19(6):6542–7.

4. Jaroff, Leon. The Man's Cancer. *Time.* April 1, 1996.

5. Yu H, Berkel H. Prostate-specific antigen (PSA) in women. *J La State Med Soc.* 1999 Apr;151(4):209–13. Review.

6. Greene KL, Albertsen PC, Babaian RJ, et al. Prostate specific antigen best practice statement: 2009 update. *J Urol.* 2009 Nov;182(5): 2232–41.

7. Vickers AJ, Till C, Tangen CM, Lilja H, Thompson IM. An empirical evaluation of guidelines on prostate-specific antigen velocity in prostate cancer detection. *J Natl Cancer Inst.* 2011 Mar 16; 103(6):462–9.

8. National Comprehensive Cancer Network. NCCN Clinical Practice Guidelines in Oncology. Prostate Cancer Early Detection. Version 2.2013.

9. Moyer VA; U.S. Preventive Services Task Force. Screening for prostate cancer: U.S. Preventive Services Task Force recommendation statement. *Ann Intern Med.* 2012 Jul 17;157(2):120–34.

10. Qaseem A, Barry MJ, Denberg TD, et al. Screening for prostate cancer: A guidance statement from the clinical guidelines committee of the American College of Physicians. *Ann Intern Med.* 2013 Apr 9.

11. Andriole GL; Crawford ED, Grubb RL, et al. Mortality results from a randomized prostate cancer screening trial. *N Engl J Med.* 2009; 360:1310–1319.

12. Andriole GL, Crawford ED, Grubb RL, Buys SS, et al.; PLCO Project Team. Mortality results from a randomized prostate-cancer screening

trial. *N Engl J Med.* 2009 Mar 26;360(13):1310–9.

13. Pinsky PF, Andriole GL, Kramer BS, Hayes RB, Prorok PC, Gohagan JK; Prostate, Lung, Colorectal and Ovarian Project Team. Prostate biopsy following a positive screen in the prostate, lung, colorectal and ovarian cancer screening trial. *J Urol.* 2005 Mar;173(3):746–50; discussion 750–1.

14. Schröder FH, Hugosson J, Roobol MJ, et al.; ERSPC Investigators. Prostate-cancer mortality at 11 years of follow-up. *N Engl J Med.* 2012 Mar 15;366(11):981–90. doi: 10.1056/NEJMoa1113135. Erratum in: N *Engl J Med.* 2012 May 31;366(22):2137.

15. Hugosson J, Carlsson S, Aus G, Bergdahl S, et al. Mortality results from the Göteborg randomised population-based prostate-cancer screening trial. *Lancet Oncol.* 2010 Aug;11(8):725–32.

16. Catalona WJ, Smith DS, Ratliff TL, et al. Measurement of prostate-specific antigen in serum as a screening test for prostate cancer. *N Engl J Med.* 1991;324:1156–1161.

17. Stephenson RA. Prostate cancer trends in the era of prostate-specific antigen. An update of incidence, mortality, and clinical factors from the SEER database. *Urol Clin North Am.* 2002 Feb;29(1):173–81.

18. Vickers AJ, Ulmert D, Sjoberg DD, et al. Strategy for detection of prostate cancer based on relation between prostate specific antigen at age 40–55 and long term risk of metastasis: case-control study. *BMJ.* 2013 Apr 15;346:f2023.

19. Carter HB, et al. Early Detection of Prostate Cancer: *AUA Guideline.* American Urological Association. 2013.

20. Hoyert DL, Xu JQ. Deaths: Preliminary data for 2011. *National Vital Statistics Reports*; vol. 61 no 6. Hyattsville, MD: National Center for Health Statistics. 2012.

21. Beckman Coulter U.S. Prostate Cancer Pivotal Study Report.

22. Lin DW, Newcomb LF, Brown EC, et al.; for the Canary Prostate Active Surveillance Study Investigators. Urinary TMPRSS2:ERG and PCA3 in an active surveillance cohort: Results from a baseline analysis in the canary prostate active surveillance study. *Clin Cancer Res.* 2013 May 1;19(9):2442–2450.

Patient Checklist

Bring this checklist with you to your next doctor's visit to get the answers you need to stay healthy.

☐ Does my family or medical history put me at a high risk for prostate cancer? _____

_____

_____

☐ Based on my age and prostate cancer risk, should I have a PSA screening and digital rectal exam? _____

_____

_____

☐ Do you recommend a PCA3 test if my PSA level comes back high?

_____

_____

☐ If my PSA test comes back high, will you retest it? _____

_____

_____

☐ What is my PSA value and what does it mean? _____

_____

_____

☐ What is my PSA density and velocity? How do you interpret these?

_____

_____

_____

Visit www.sprypubprostate.com to download a printable checklist.

CHAPTER THREE

Redefining Prostate Cancer

One Man's Story

Sid is an 83-year-old award-winning writer who was diagnosed with a Gleason 8 high-risk prostate cancer. Because of his age, the urologist who diagnosed his tumor was reluctant to give him the treatment most likely to cure his cancer—a radical prostatectomy surgery. Life expectancy tables predicted that, on average, men Sid's age live only another 6 or 7 years, so on the face of things, the urologist was choosing a statistically safe option. But as a relatively healthy man with a still thriving career, Sid found this assumption ridiculous. He went in search of a second opinion from Dr. Lepor.

After reviewing Sid's history and biopsy results, they discussed his age and the associated surgical risks and benefits. Dr. Lepor told Sid about a conversation he had with a mentor back in medical school. When asked about surgical treatment for prostate cancer in men older than 70, the mentor replied: "Operate on someone age 70 or older only if their parents are available to sign the consent form."

Without missing a beat, Sid offered to get his mother's blessing at her 106th birthday party, which was taking place the following month. His 96- and 101-year-old aunts were also scheduled to attend.

Clearly Sid was not your typical 83-year-old, driving home the fact that "one size does not fit all" when it comes to prostate cancer. Given his general good health and the longevity in his family history, another 20 years of life would not be unheard of. So denying him the surgery to remove a high-risk prostate cancer was very likely to cut his life expectancy. Recognizing the individual nature of this disease and the odds in Sid's favor, Dr. Lepor agreed to schedule the surgery for the next week on one condition—that Sid sends him a picture of himself and his mother at her birthday celebration.

Prostate Cancer Is Not a Death Sentence

Prostate cancer is the most common type of cancer diagnosed in men, and it continues to grow in incidence. In 2009, 206,640 American men were diagnosed with the condition, and for 2013, the American Cancer Society estimates 238,590 will receive a diagnosis.[1,2] Yet there are 2.5 million men living in the United States who are prostate cancer survivors.

Incidence of Prostate Cancer Diagnosis

One in six men will be diagnosed with prostate cancer in their lifetime. The number of diagnoses grows steadily after age 40. An estimated 8.54% of men will develop cancer of the prostate between age 50 and 70. Statistics show that incidence peaks during the ages of 70 to 74, when 977 out of every 100,000 men develop prostate cancer.[3]

Death Rate from Prostate Cancer

Considering the high incidence and prevalence of prostate cancer, the death rate is actually remarkably low. For every 100,000 U.S. adult male deaths, 23.6 of those are attributable to prostate cancer, a rate that has been decreasing since the early 1990s. Prostate cancer is a leading cause of male cancer death, second only to lung cancer in men. Yet it also offers men some of the best survival odds, with a 5-year relative survival of 99.2%. This means when you average survival rates among men with all types and stages of prostate cancer, 99.2% of men will live at least five years post-diagnosis. The 10-year survival rate is almost as impressive at 98%. For localized prostate cancers (those that have not spread past the prostate), the 5-year survival rate is even better—100% (see figure 5).[4]

Estimated number of new cases 2013 – 238,590

Estimated number of deaths 2013 – 29,720 (10%)

Probability (%) of developing invasive prostate cancer during selected age intervals (2007–2009)

Age 40–59 2.68% (1 in 37)

Age 60–69 6.78% (1 in 15)

Age 70 & older 12.06% (1 in 8)

Survival rates by stage

Local stage (Stages I and II)

Regional stage (Stages III and IV that haven't spread to distant parts of the body, such as T4 tumors and cancers that have spread to nearby lymph nodes (N1).)

Distant stage (the rest of the stage IV cancers)

5-year relative survival by stage at the time of diagnosis

Stage	5-year relative survival rate
local	nearly 100%
regional	nearly 100%
distant	28%

Cancer incidence by race & ethnicity (per 100,000)

African-American 228.7

Caucasian 141.0

Hispanic/Latino 124.9

American-Indian or Alaska Native 98.8

Asian American or Pacific Islander 77.2

Figure 5. Prostate cancer information. Source: American Cancer Society, Surveillance Research 2013.

If prostate cancer is the second leading cause of cancer death, why do they say men die *with* it and not *from* it?

A common adage in the world of prostate cancer is that men die *with* the disease, not *from* it. One of the reasons we say this is the nature of the cancer itself. An estimated 70% of diagnosed prostate cancers are considered low risk with an excellent prognosis.[5] Even those considered medium or high risk are highly treatable. And in the modern age of PSA testing and advanced imaging, we are much more likely to find these low-risk cancers.

We've also found there are cancers that we never detect, or preferably should not detect, known as "autopsy cancers." These are cancers found during autopsy in men who have died from non-cancer related reasons. They develop late in life and cause no problem. Some studies show that 30% of prostates obtained from men over the age of 50 upon autopsy will have some prostate cancer.[6] So statistically, the overwhelming majority of men with prostate cancer will not die from their cancers but with them.

Prostate Cancer: A Spectrum of Diseases

Prostate cancer runs the gamut from slow-growing low-risk tumors that may cause a man no adverse effects in his lifetime to aggressive late-stage cancer that has spread to other organs and tissues. Fortunately, around 70% of diagnosed prostate cancers are of the early-stage type. The different stages and risk levels of cancers are discussed in detail in chapter 4.

Slow Growing to Diffuse Metastasis

Early-stage prostate cancers are typically treated by surgically removing or destroying the entire prostate gland. Focal therapy or ablation is another investigational option where only the visible cancer seen on imaging is destroyed. Some low-risk cancers may not require any treatment or may just need to be closely monitored through regular testing (a treatment known as "active surveillance").

Metastatic prostate cancer is cancer that has spread from the prostate to other parts of the body, such as the bones, liver, or lungs. It spreads when prostate cancer grows outside of the prostate gland after invading the lymphatic system and/or blood vessels. Cancer cells can then travel these routes to reach other parts of the body.

Is my prostate cancer curable?

If you have a cancer that is completely confined to the prostate, we can say with fair certainty that we can remove or destroy it with surgery, radiation, or ablation. Now by the time a cancer has metastasized to other sites outside of the prostate, we have certain ways we can arrest the disease for a time period with hormonal therapy. We also have chemotherapy and immune therapy that may extend life months or even years once the cancer becomes hormone insensitive. But these cancers cannot be cured by any treatments currently available to us. That is why it is so important to find and evaluate cancers before they metastasize.

Treatment Priorities: Cure vs. Quality of Life

When deciding on a treatment, men and their doctors need to weigh the benefits of treatment against any adverse impact they will have on a man's quality of life. Surgery and other treatments can have side effects that can affect a man's sexual performance and that can cause unpleasant urinary and bowel symptoms. While for many men these side effects are temporary, they can be long lasting and may not resolve completely. Depending on their age, health, and lifestyle considerations, some men may prefer to forego these treatments to maintain their quality of life.

For Dr. Lepor's patient Sid, surgical treatment was a choice that made sense. Even though he did not fit the profile of a typical surgical candidate in terms of age, Sid's health and family history made him a good candidate. He felt he could cope with some temporary urinary issues following the surgery, and that any potential long-term sexual side effects would not have a major impact on his quality of life. And, of course, the prospect of living another 15 years or longer was a huge benefit.

Causes and Risk Factors

Doctors and researchers still do not know exactly what causes prostate cancer. We do know that mutations in our DNA—the genetic material that contains the instructions for cell growth—are what triggers cancerous changes in the prostate. Some mutations are inherited at birth and others occur during a man's lifetime.

We also know that certain factors can increase your prostate cancer risk. Some of these, such as age, race, and family history, we have no influence over. But we may be able to do something about other environmental factors.

Age

While prostate cancer can occur in men of any age, the risk increases as you age. An estimated 60% of prostate cancers are found in men over age 65, and 97% are diagnosed in men over age 50.[7] The condition is extremely rare in men under age 40.

Race

African-American men are at a higher risk for developing prostate cancer. The incidence of prostate cancer is 70% higher in African-American men than in whites. American-Indian and Native Alaskan men have the lowest incidence of prostate cancer among American men.[8]

Family History

Men who have a brother or father diagnosed with prostate cancer are twice as likely to develop the disease. Having a brother with prostate cancer increases risk more than having a father with it. The more first-degree relatives who have the disease, the higher the risk. And having male relatives who were diagnosed with prostate cancer before age 65 also increases a man's risk.[9] Second-degree relatives with prostate cancer, such as an uncle or grandfather, also raise risk, although less so than fathers and brothers.[10]

My brother has prostate cancer. What can I do to prevent prostate cancer?

First and foremost, you should be screened for prostate cancer beginning at age 40 given your family risk. Catching any cancer early on and treating it appropriately is the best way to manage prostate cancer successfully. As far as prevention goes, healthy lifestyle habits such as regular exercise, cutting out tobacco, and eating a variety of fruits and vegetables will help you maintain your overall health, although there is no direct proven link to prostate cancer prevention. Chapter 1 of this book has more specific recommendations on living healthy for you and your prostate.

In several large trials, the 5-alpha-reductase-inhibitor (5-ARI) drugs finasteride and dutasteride, which have been used to treat men with BPH, were found to lower the relative risk of developing low-risk prostate cancers (Gleason 6 or lower) by 26% in men undergoing regular prostate cancer screening.[11] However, use of the drugs has been associated with a statistical increase in the number of high-risk prostate cancers (Gleason 8–10). For this reason, the FDA has not approved these as chemopreventive (cancer prevention) drugs.[12]

If you take 5-ARI drugs for BPH or for male pattern hair loss (Propecia is also a 5-ARI drug), talk to your doctor about your prostate cancer risk and an appropriate screening schedule. Be aware that the regular use of 5-ARI drugs also artificially lowers PSA results by about 50%, so any PSA screening should be interpreted with this in mind.

Diet

A diet high in dairy may increase your risk of prostate cancer according to some studies.[13] Grilled and well-done red meats have also been associated with increased risk.[14,15]

On the other hand, cruciferous vegetables (e.g., broccoli), lycopene-rich tomatoes, fish, and soy have been linked to a *reduced* risk of certain types of prostate cancers. Adding these foods to your diet may be helpful if you aren't eating them already.[16]

Lifestyle

Where you live may also play a role in your prostate cancer risk. Long-term studies have found that men who live at latitudes above 40 degrees (e.g., Portland, Oregon; Minneapolis, Minnesota; Boston, Massachusetts) have a higher risk of mortality from prostate cancer. Researchers theorize that this may be due to the lower amounts of total annual sunlight in these regions, an important contributor to vitamin D intake.[17]

There are many other environmental and lifestyle factors that have been linked to a potential increase in prostate cancer, but many require further long-term study to prove a link. Some of these have enough substantial research behind them to make them worth calling out here:

- **Obesity**—Obese men may be more likely to develop more aggressive prostate cancers.[18]
- **Pesticide Exposure**—Certain pesticides have also been linked to aggressive prostate cancer.[19]
- **Sedentary Behavior**—Studies have linked a lack of regular exercise to increased prostate cancer risk.[20]

Is there a relationship between BPH and prostate cancer?

Some men worry that benign prostatic hyperplasia can later develop into prostate cancer. There is no known relationship between these two conditions. However, the risk of both increases as men age. BPH is rare before age 40, but occurs in half of men over age 50, and up to 90% of men age 70 and older. Similarly, your prostate cancer risk also increases exponentially after age 40. But again, the two conditions are not directly related, and if you have BPH it does not mean you will also develop prostate cancer.

Symptoms of Prostate Cancer

Early-stage prostate cancer usually has no symptoms, which is why screening is such an important tool. But as a prostate tumor grows or develops into a more aggressive cancer, a man may experience one or more of the following symptoms:
- weak or interrupted urine stream
- urinary urgency (feeling like you have to go all the time)
- difficulty starting or stopping urine flow
- frequent urination, especially at night
- pain or burning with urination
- blood in the urine
- hip, spine, rib, or other bone pain
- weight loss
- anemia

It's important to remember that many of these urinary symptoms can occur with non-cancerous conditions such as BPH and prostatitis. Bone pain is rare and only occurs with later-stage prostate cancers that have metastasized (spread) to the bones.

Putting It All Together

Sid underwent outpatient radical prostatectomy surgery with no complications. Two weeks later, he was back working on his latest writing project. The following month, Dr. Lepor received a photo of a smiling 83-year-old Sid and his 106-year-old mother blowing out birthday candles. He keeps it on his office wall as a visible reminder of the uniqueness of every prostate cancer patient.

References

1. U.S. Cancer Statistics Working Group. *United States Cancer Statistics: 1999–2009 Incidence and Mortality Web-based Report*. Atlanta (GA): Department of Health and Human Services, Centers for Disease Control and Prevention, and National Cancer Institute; 2013. Available at: http://www.cdc.gov/uscs.

2. American Cancer Society. *Cancer Facts & Figures 2013*. Atlanta, Ga: American Cancer Society; 2013.

3. Howlader N, Noone AM, Krapcho M, et al. (eds). *SEER Cancer Statistics Review, 1975-2009* (Vintage 2009 Populations), National Cancer Institute. Bethesda, MD, http://seer.cancer.gov/csr/1975_2009_pops09/, based on November 2011 SEER data submission, posted to the SEER web site, 2012.

4. American Cancer Society. *Cancer Facts & Figures 2013*. Atlanta, GA: American Cancer Society; 2013.

5. Hayes JH, Ollendorf DA, Pearson SD, et al. Active surveillance compared with initial treatment for men with low-risk prostate cancer: a decision analysis. *JAMA*. 2010 Dec 1;304(21):2373–80.

6. Scardino PT. Early detection of prostate cancer. *Urol Clin North Am*. 1989 Nov;16(4):635–55. Review.

7. American Cancer Society. *Cancer Facts & Figures 2013*. Atlanta, GA: American Cancer Society; 2013.

8. Centers for Disease Control. Division of Cancer Prevention and Control. National Center for Chronic Disease Prevention and Health Promotion Division. Prostate Cancer Incidence Rates by Race and Ethnicity, U.S., 1999–2009.

9. Zeegers MP, Jellema A, Ostrer H. Empiric risk of prostate carcinoma for relatives of patients with prostate carcinoma: a meta-analysis. *Cancer* 2003 Apr 15;97(8):1894–903.

10. National Cancer Institute: PDQ® *Genetics of Prostate Cancer*. Bethesda, MD: National Cancer Institute. Available at: http://cancer.gov/cancertopics/pdq/genetics/prostate/HealthProfessional. Accessed 04/21/2013.

11. Wilt TJ, MacDonald R, Hagerty K, Schellhammer P, Kramer BS.

5-alpha-reductase inhibitors for prostate cancer prevention. *Cochrane Database of Systematic Reviews 2008*, Issue 2. Art. No.: CD007091. DOI: 10.1002/14651858.CD007091.

12. FDA Drug Safety Communication: 5-alpha reductase inhibitors (5-ARIs) may increase the risk of a more serious form of prostate cancer. 2011 June 9.

13. Song Y, Chavarro JE, Cao Y, et al. Whole milk intake is associated with prostate cancer-specific mortality among U.S. male physicians. *J Nutr*. 2013 Feb;143(2):189–96.

14. Punnen S, Hardin J, Cheng I, Klein EA, Witte JS. Impact of meat consumption, preparation, and mutagens on aggressive prostate ancer. *PLoS One*. 2011;6(11):e27711.

15. Major JM, Cross AJ, Watters JL, Hollenbeck AR, Graubard BI, Sinha R. Patterns of meat intake and risk of prostate cancer among African-Americans in a large prospective study. *Cancer Causes Control*. 2011 Dec;22(12):1691–8.

16. Leitzmann MF, Rohrmann S. Risk factors for the onset of prostatic cancer: age, location, and behavioral correlates. *Clin Epidemiol*. 2012;4:1–11.

17. Schwartz GG, Hanchette CL. UV, latitude, and spatial trends in prostate cancer mortality: all sunlight is not the same (United States). *Cancer Causes Control*. 2006 Oct;17(8):1091–101.

18. Allott EH, Masko EM, Freedland SJ. Obesity and prostate cancer: weighing the evidence. *Eur Urol*. 2013 May;63(5):800–9.

19. Koutros S, Beane Freeman LE, Lubin JH, et al. Risk of total and aggressive prostate cancer and pesticide use in the Agricultural Health Study. *Am J Epidemiol*. 2013 Jan 1;177(1):59–74.

20. Lynch BM. Sedentary behavior and cancer: a systematic review of the literature and proposed biological mechanisms. *Cancer Epidemiol Biomarkers Prev*. 2010 Nov;19(11):2691–709.

Patient Checklist

Bring this checklist with you to your next doctor's visit to get the answers you need to stay healthy.

☐ I do not have prostate cancer. Does anything in my personal, health, or family history increase my risk of getting it? Should I be screened, and if so, how and when? _____

_____

_____

_____

_____

_____

☐ I do not have prostate cancer, but one or more relatives have had it. Am I at increased risk and what precautions should I take?

_____

_____

_____

_____

_____

☐ I have prostate cancer. Should other men in my family (brothers, father, sons) undergo regular screening now that they are at higher risk? If so, what and when? _____

_____

_____

_____

_____

_____

_____

Visit www.sprypubprostate.com to download a printable checklist.

CHAPTER FOUR

Making the Diagnosis: Imaging and Biopsy

One Man's Story

Jack is a 62-year-old married man who is visiting the doctor for his annual physical. An avid runner and former athlete, Jack is in excellent physical condition and reports feeling better today than he did in his 40s. When he turned 50, Jack got his first PSA test at the recommendation of his doctor (and following American Cancer Society guidelines). He has followed up with annual testing ever since.

Several days after his physical, Jack gets a call from the doctor. This is the fourth year in a row that his PSA levels have risen significantly (2.1, 2.7, 4.0, 5.5 ng/mL). Last year, Jack's doctor had ordered a transrectal ultrasound (TRUS)-guided biopsy of his prostate. That biopsy took 12 random core samples of Jack's prostate, and the results came back negative for prostate cancer. His doctor is concerned about this continued rise in PSA, especially with no other symptoms of prostate infection or inflammation. After some discussion, Jack and his doctor agree that he should go in for a multiparametric MRI to get a closer look at his prostate and biopsy any areas of concern.

Imaging methods such as ultrasound and MRI allow us to get a closer and more accurate look at the prostate. With these tools, we can find smaller tumors and also target areas of concern for biopsy. Biopsy involves sampling tissue from the prostate in order to confirm the presence of cancer and analyze the cancerous tissue to establish the level of risk it poses for spreading.

The Biopsy Decision

If your doctor feels a mass during DRE, biopsy is a fairly straight-forward process. The mass can and should be easily targeted, sampled, and tested for the presence of prostate cancer. But the vast majority of prostate biopsies today are on men with a normal DRE and an elevated PSA test. In the absence of a clear tumor target, most urologists biopsy with a technique that randomly samples different areas throughout the prostate seeking a clinically significant cancer. This is known as transrectal ultrasound (TRUS)-guided random core biopsy. However, more accurate (yet less widespread) imaging techniques for finding cancer are now available and discussed later in this chapter.

Before suggesting biopsy, your doctor will repeat your PSA test to ensure there was no laboratory error. He may also perform additional laboratory tests, such as the PCA3 (described in detail in chapter 2). Other conditions that raise PSA levels, such as prostatitis and BPH, should be ruled out with confidence before a biopsy is recommended.

Risks and Benefits

Biopsy is an invasive procedure and carries a risk of infection, al-though antibiotic treatment minimizes that risk. And there is always a chance that a random core biopsy will not detect a clinically signif-icant cancer if the core samples that are taken miss cancerous tissue.

The main benefit, of course, is that biopsy can identify those cancers that, without treatment, could be life threatening. And as more accurate imaging techniques are put into use, such as mpMRI, doctors are able to more precisely target clinically significant cancers.

My PSA is abnormal, should I get a biopsy?

Biopsies are invasive procedures that can cause side effects, discomfort, and anxiety. And as discussed earlier, the PSA is not a foolproof test. Before ordering a biopsy, your doctor should do some additional investigation. First of all, the abnormal PSA should be repeated to ensure there was no laboratory error. Second, your doctor will try to rule out other causes of an elevated PSA through physical exam, other laboratory tests, and your medical history. Finally, additional tests such as PCA3 and mpMRI can be very helpful in determining whether prostate cancer is likely, so talk to your doctor about whether or not these tests are a good choice for you.

TRUS-Guided Biopsies

The current standard of care in the United States is to biopsy random sections of the prostate for cancerous tissue under ultrasound guidance (or sound waves), a method that can be a bit like searching for a needle in a haystack in terms of accuracy (see figure 6). While TRUS-guided biopsy targets the areas of the prostate statistically most likely to contain cancers, it can miss those cancers that occur in non-sampled areas.

The prostate is comprised of peripheral and transition zones. Since the majority of cancers develop in the peripheral zone, early TRUS-guided biopsies were directed into the peripheral zone of the prostate and randomly yet systematically sampled six tissue cores.

A TRUS-guided biopsy is usually performed in the urologist's office. There is some preparation required before the procedure. You will be asked to give yourself an enema the morning of the biopsy to clear the rectum. Your doctor will also prescribe antibiotics prior to the procedure to be taken the day before and the day of the biopsy. Aspirin and nonsteroidal anti-inflammatory drugs (NSAIDs) should not be taken a week prior to the procedure. In addition, if you take any anticoagulant drugs for heart conditions, you may be advised to stop them a week before, as well. You should always check with the prescribing doctor before discontinuing a medicine, even temporarily.

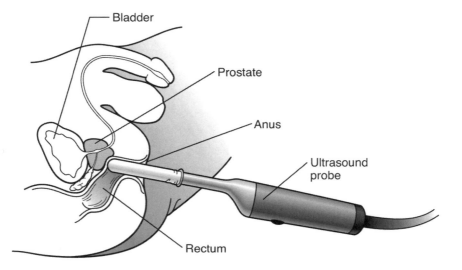

Figure 6. TRUS-guided biopsy procedure. An ultrasound probe is placed in the rectum and used to guide collection of multiple prostate tissue specimens for analysis.

Before the procedure begins, your doctor will administer a local anesthetic to numb the prostate area. An ultrasound probe about a half-inch wide is inserted into the rectum and used to visualize the prostate and guide the biopsy device. Samples are then taken with the biopsy needle, and the whole procedure is usually complete in 15 minutes. The biopsy procedure causes relatively minor pain as the biopsies are being taken.

12-Core Random Biopsy: The Current Standard

The first TRUS-guided procedures used a standard 6 core samples for biopsy. But in the late 1990s, experts (including Dr. Lepor, one of the authors of this book) found that 6 random biopsies did not adequately sample the prostate.[1] A TRUS-guided random systematic biopsy technique with 12 tissue cores identified 30% more cancers than the 6-core version. Shortly thereafter, most urologists started to use biopsy protocols that obtained between 10 and 12 tissue cores (see figure 7).

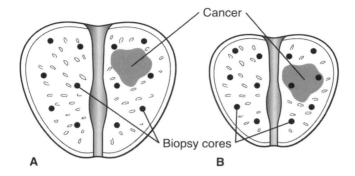

Figure 7. Prostate zones for 12-core biopsy. A standard 12-core biopsy can miss cancer in a larger prostate gland simply because there is more tissue to sample than in a smaller prostate. In sample B, cancer is detected in two biopsy samples but missed in sample A, even though the cancers are similar in size.

Potential Side Effects

Mild discomfort in the perineum (the space between the scrotum and rectum) may occur for a few days following TRUS-guided biopsy. The most serious risk of prostate biopsy is a blood-borne systemic infection. Over the past few years, there has been an increasing percentage of men who develop serious systemic infections following a biopsy.[2] The initial symptoms are usually fever and chills. In these cases, bacteria resistant to the quinolones (antibacterial drugs) gain access to the blood stream, creating a potentially life-threatening infection. Quinolone-resistant bacteria are becoming more common due to widespread use of the antibiotics in the general community. In order to decrease the incidence of these infections, it is now common for a urologist to inject the patient with a broad-spectrum antibiotic immediately prior to a TRUS-guided biopsy.

The other major complication following TRUS-guided biopsy is bleeding. This is usually controlled by applying pressure with the examining finger. If severe, a small suture may be required. Blood may also be encountered in the urine or semen. When bleeding into the urine is extensive, clots may develop and impede bladder emptying.

In these rare cases, a urinary catheter may be required to facilitate urination for a few days. Men are asked to urinate after the procedure and prior to leaving the office to ensure that the bladder is emptying. Blood in the semen is not harmful. Over time, the semen will return to its normal color and consistency. While blood in the semen is resolving, no limitations or precautions on sexual activity are required.

Are twelve tissue cores enough to find cancer?

The average volume of the prostate glands of men undergoing biopsy averages about 40 cm^3 (range 20 cm^3 to >100 cm^3). Twelve cores of tissue still represent a very small sampling of the total prostate. In addition, there are some cancers that originate in the transition (central) zone of the prostate, and this region is not routinely sampled as part of a 12-core biopsy. Therefore, while better than the old 6-core method, many cancers can still be missed by a 12-core TRUS-guided biopsy.

Saturation Biopsy

A saturation biopsy is designed to sample the entire prostate gland (see figure 8). Using a grid system, between 50 and 100 tissue core samples are taken from the prostate (the exact number depends on the size and volume of the gland). This procedure is performed under general or spinal anesthesia and is associated with greater discomfort and bleeding than TRUS-guided 12-core random biopsy.

Saturation biopsy should be reserved for those men who have had one or more negative TRUS-guided biopsies and a progressively rising PSA. In some cases where focal therapy is being considered, a saturation biopsy will help find those areas containing clinically significant cancers.

Common side effects from saturation biopsy include pain and urinary problems, although these usually decrease with time.[3] In addition, the procedure may make it more difficult to perform radical prostatectomy surgery in the future if one is needed.

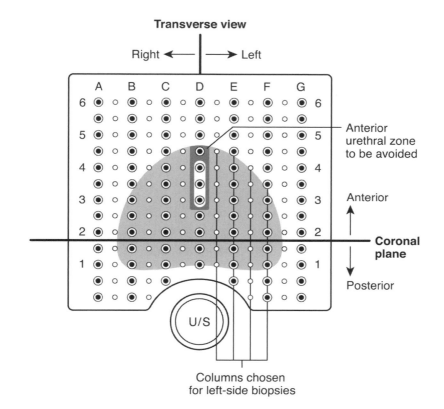

Figure 8. Prostate gland as seen by transrectal ultrasound (U/S) probe during a saturation biopsy. A catheter is in place to readily identify the prostatic urethra that must be avoided to prevent injury.

Multiparametric MRI: A Game Changer

Magnetic resonance imaging (MRI) was first used in the mid-1980s to locate prostate tumors.[4] But the process at that time was imperfect; it only detected larger tumors and it also required that the patient hold a coil in the rectum for 30 minutes.

But within the past decade, a newer MRI technology has been developed that can detect earlier-stage tumors and does not require use of an endorectal coil. This technology, known as multiparametric MRI (mpMRI), has revolutionized the detection of prostate cancer.

mpMRI can detect prostate cancer in three different ways. First of all, we look at *angiogenesis*, which is new blood vessel formation. We know that tumor tissue has increased nutrient demands compared to surrounding tissue. The body supports that increased nutrient need by building new blood vessels to feed the tumor tissue, and we often can see that activity on MRI. Not only can we see it, we also know that this immature bed of vascular tissue in the area of tumor has leaky capillaries. So we know that blood will flow very quickly into that tumor tissue due to the increased vascularity, as well as wash out very quickly. This is known as "wash in/wash out."

Secondly, we look for something called *diffusion restriction*. MRI essentially looks at protons and water, of which the body is mostly composed. With normal tissue, the cells of the body have enough space around them for water to flow freely. In tumor tissue, the cells start to cluster more tightly together because they're dividing very quickly and do not have time to space apart. All those cells clustered together form a barrier to water movement and cell membranes restrict water flow. This is called restricted diffusion. We can actually create an image with the MRI in areas that show very slow water movement, which indicates a tumor.

The third and final way we look at tumors is the original way MRI was used, called *T2-weighted MRI*. We look at the outer portion of the prostate gland. A normal prostate has a lot of water in it, which looks very white or bright on MRI. We know that tumor tissue will look dark on that particular sequence in the peripheral zone or outer part of the prostate gland. Any black or dark areas in those areas of white in the outer part of the prostate gland are suspicious for tumor.

When we analyze the MRI with all three of these parameters, it allows us to examine every part of the prostate gland to see if it's abnormal in all three, one out of three, or two out of three parameters. Something that's abnormal on all three parameters is going to most likely be cancer, while something that's only positive on the dynamic contrast enhancement parameter, or angiogenesis, is going to just show inflammation or possibly a low-grade cancer. So many times we can say that something is most likely prostatitis and not tumor, and if it is tumor it's likely not going to be aggressive.

mpMRI before Biopsy

We believe that mpMRI is going to revolutionize the diagnosis and treatment of prostate cancer screening, detection, and treatment. Today, there is a small yet increasing number of experts who recommend mpMRI before performing an initial prostate biopsy. At the Smilow Comprehensive Prostate Cancer Center and Sperling Prostate Center, urologists and radiologists work collaboratively, and an mpMRI is obtained in all men prior to undergoing the prostate biopsy.[5] It allows us to hone in on potential targets that have a high probability of representing a cancer rather than the "pin the tail on the donkey" approach of TRUS-guided random sample core biopsy.

Recent studies suggest that in regions where the mpMRI is negative, clinically significant disease on biopsy is rarely found.[6,7,8] In other words, it seems to accurately rule out the presence of clinically significant prostate cancers. Therefore, it may not be necessary to randomly biopsy areas of the prostate that are negative on MRI. This approach requires more study and further validation.

We believe using mpMRI before biopsy is an important strategy for screening and detection of prostate cancer. mpMRI selectively identifies those potentially lethal cancers while minimizing over-detection and over-treatment of clinically insignificant disease. Ultimately, widespread use could greatly decrease the number of men undergoing unnecessary prostate biopsy.

Should an MRI be performed prior to a prostate biopsy?

If mpMRI is available in your area, ask your urologist if it's possible to get one prior to your prostate biopsy. It is currently the best possible way to pick up clinically significant tumors while at the same time avoiding over-treatment and over-diagnosis of very-low-grade cancer. Keep in mind that men with certain types of pacemakers and other implanted medical devices may not be candidates for MRI, as metal cannot be used in an MRI machine. If you have these devices, have a discussion with the radiologist about whether or not you are eligible for mpMRI.

In-gantry MRI Biopsy

Some facilities have the capabilities to do biopsies inside the MRI scanner. This is called *in-gantry MRI-guided biopsy of the prostate*. As the MRI images the prostate, the radiologist is able to put a biopsy needle directly into the suspected tumor tissue to sample it (unlike the random sample approach of TRUS-guided biopsy). In addition, it allows the radiologist to image the needle within the tumor itself and document that the lesion was accurately sampled.

This can be particularly helpful for finding and biopsying cancer in the anterior portion of the prostate gland, as TRUS-guided biopsies usually can't sample that area appropriately and often miss these tumors. The apex of the prostate also tends to be undersampled with TRUS-guided biopsy due to its proximity to the delicate urethra. The in-gantry MRI approach allows the radiologist to clearly visualize the tumor and the urethra, therefore potentially not missing as many tumors in the apex of the prostate gland. And again, because the mpMRI preferentially picks up cancers of clinical significance, unnecessary biopsies may be avoided.

Unfortunately, very few U.S. radiologists are currently trained to perform in-gantry biopsy. The Sperling Prostate Center (see appendix A) is one of the few centers in the United States currently performing this procedure. Dr. Sperling trained in the Netherlands to learn the technology. Even fewer radiologists have enough experience with prostate cancer to manage potential complications of prostate biopsy and be familiar with the nuances of disease biology. While collaborative radiologist/urologist relationships do exist, such as the one we have, they are the exception rather than the rule. And with over one million biopsies performed annually in the United States, in-gantry biopsy is just not an option for many patients.

Co-registration Biopsy

A co-registration biopsy involves targeting a tumor with an mpMRI, then using that information to perform the biopsy under TRUS guidance. There are two types of co-registration biopsy: cognitive and three-dimensional (3-D).

Cognitive Co-registration

Most urologists who are already skilled in TRUS-guided biopsy can perform cognitive co-registration. The urologist uses information from a previously completed mpMRI to pinpoint an area of the prostate for biopsy. The urologist then mentally superimposes the mpMRI on the TRUS image and targets what he believes is the cancerous tissue on the ultrasound. This technique is more likely to have a positive result when the suspected cancerous area is large.

3-D Co-registration Biopsy

Three-dimensional co-registration biopsy is a new technology that uses computer software to three-dimensionally co-register, or super-impose, the area identified by the mpMRI onto a TRUS image. While several co-registration devices are under development, the greatest experience is with the Artemis system with ProFuse software, developed by Eigen. First, a radiologist runs an mpMRI to find any areas of the prostate with clinically significant cancers. Then during a trans-rectal ultrasound, the device superimposes the mpMRI onto the real-time TRUS images. Through this combined imaging technique, the urologist is guided to the exact target for biopsy.

There are a few potential drawbacks to co-registration. If the time between mpMRI and biopsy is too long, the prostate gland can change shape in the interim, causing a misregistration and the potential for a tumor to be missed. The ultrasound device can also deform the prostate gland and make the registration process inaccurate. Newer versions of fusion are currently under development that will more accurately register the ultrasound and MRI images and account for gland contour differences.

New York University Langone Medical Center, where Dr. Lepor practices, was one of the first prostate cancer treatment facilities to acquire the Artemis ProFuse system and more than 300 biopsies have been performed there using this new 3-D technology. Preliminary data as of March 2013 indicate that random biopsies of regions of the prostate that appear normal on MRI rarely detect clinically significant cancers. This makes a further case for a biopsy strategy that uses mpMRI or a 3-D co-registration system to target clinically significant cancers.

Understanding Your Biopsy Results

Once your biopsy is complete, the tissue samples are sent to a pathologist for microscopic review and analysis. Several days to a week following your biopsy, the pathology results should be available. Your doctor's office should alert you when the results are available so you can review them together, but it's a good idea to ask at the time of the biopsy what system is in place to get you the results (and when). You should also ask that a copy of the pathology report be sent to you for your records.

If your pathology report reveals cancer, it will contain detailed information about the stage and type of prostate cancer involved that will help to guide you and your doctor in deciding on appropriate treatment. This includes the Gleason score.

Gleason Score

The Gleason score is used to categorize the risk level of a man's prostate cancer. It's named after Dr. Donald Gleason, the pathologist who developed the system in the 1960s. Gleason scores are based on the appearance of prostate cancer under the microscope. A pathologist examines the cell patterns in the biopsy tissue samples and assigns a grade. Tissue patterns can be rated anywhere from closely resembling normal tissue (grade 1) to highly aggressive and invasive cancer (grade 5). The pathologist identifies the two most prominent patterns in the sample with the highest grades and adds those two values together, resulting in the Gleason score. A Gleason score can range from 2 to

10; most cancers will range from 6 to 8. The higher the Gleason score, the more aggressive the cancer (see table 1) and the higher the risk it will spread.

Table 1. Interpreting Risk from the Gleason Score

Risk	Gleason Score
Low	6
Intermediate	7
High	8–10

Because just one point can mean the difference between a low- and intermediate-grade cancer, or between an intermediate- and high-grade cancer, the accuracy of a biopsy has a major influence on how accurate the Gleason score is. One study of 222 men who underwent random core systematic biopsy found that 46% of biopsy results underestimated the actual Gleason grade of the cancer when the prostate was removed during later radical prostatectomy surgery and the entire specimen was examined by a pathologist.[9]

Some urologists may use a risk stratification system known as the D'Amico system to assess the aggressiveness of your prostate cancer. The D'Amico system calculates risk based on the Gleason score, the PSA, and tumor stage (see table 2).[10]

Table 2. D'Amico Risk Stratification System

Risk	Gleason Score	Tumor Stage	PSA
Low	≤6	T1c–T2a	≤10 ng/mL
Intermediate	7	T2b	10–20 ng/mL
High	≥8	T2c	>20 ng/mL

My PSA keeps rising and two biopsies are negative ... should I get a third biopsy?

Because random biopsies have the potential to miss clinically significant cancers, repeat biopsies are sometimes necessary. This is especially true when PSA continues to rise despite negative biopsies. In a case like yours, additional tests such as PCA3 and mpMRI would be useful in more accurately assessing cancer risk and targeted additional biopsies. Speak with your doctor about these options.

Tumor Size and Staging

If you get a random core biopsy or a saturation biopsy, your pathology report should indicate how many cores were taken in the biopsy sample and how many of these tested positive for cancer cells. Your biopsy report is one indicator of tumor risk.

The clinical stage of the tumor reflects the volume of cancer detected by DRE and whether the cancer appears to be contained within the gland or has spread beyond the prostate capsule.[11] T1c is the most commonly diagnosed clinical stage of prostate cancer. The stages of prostate cancer are listed in table 3 and illustrated in figure 9.

Table 3. Clinical Stages of Prostate Cancer

Clinical Stage	Finding
T1	Tumor can't be felt on DRE or seen on radiology tests.
T1a*	Tumor (cancerous tissue) found in <5% of the pathology sample.
T1b*	Tumor found in >5% of pathology sample.
T1c	Tumor found with needle biopsy after elevated PSA test result.
T2	Tumor felt on DRE or seen on imaging tests; confined to the prostate.
T2a	Tumor is felt in less than half of one lobe (or side) of the prostate.
T2b	Tumor is felt in more than half of one lobe (side) of the prostate.
T2c	Tumor is felt on both lobes (sides) of the prostate.
T3	Cancer extends beyond the capsule of the prostate.
T4	Cancer has invaded other tissues and organs surrounding the prostate (e.g., bladder, rectum, pelvic wall).

T1a and T1b tumors are typically found by accident during prostate surgery for other conditions such as BPH.

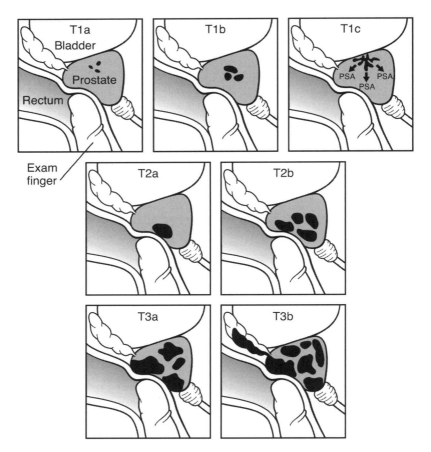

Figure 9. Types of prostate cancer tumors by clinical stage.

Do I need a CT scan or bone scan to assess my prostate cancer?

For men with high-risk disease, metastasis to the lymph nodes and skeletal system is more common. In these men, abdominal/pelvic CT or MRI and a bone scan should be performed to look for any cancer spread before deciding on a treatment course.

Histological Types

Histology refers to the microscopic structure of cells and tissue. Almost all prostate cancers have a histological type of adenocarcinoma. A small minority (under 5%) are rarer cancers, including small cell neuroendocrine tumors, sarcomas, and lymphomas. Your biopsy report should indicate your histological type.

There are two pre-cancerous, or pre-malignant, conditions that can show up on biopsy—high-grade prostatic intraepithelial neoplasia (HGPIN) and atypical small acinar proliferation (ASAP). Acini are the tiny sacs that produce the fluid for ejaculation. Because both of these conditions can co-exist or advance to cancer, they need to be followed closely with PSA tests and potential re-biopsy.

Putting It All Together

Jack undergoes an mpMRI, which uncovers a suspicious area that requires further investigation. His doctor also orders a PCA3 test and the result is 65, well above the upper limit of normal of 25. With these results in hand, Jack's doctor recommends a targeted biopsy. Jack goes to the Smilow Comprehensive Prostate Cancer Center and undergoes a 3-D co-registration biopsy, which reveals a Gleason 7 cancer, something his previous two random sample biopsies missed.

The following month, Jack opts to have radical prostatectomy surgery. He experiences some temporary urinary leakage and erection problems, but both return to normal within months. At his one-year follow-up, Jack is feeling great. The PSA level is undetectable (<0.01), and he is back on his running schedule and awaiting the birth of his first grandchild.

References

1. Levine MA, Ittman M, Melamed J, Lepor H. Two consecutive sets of transrectal ultrasound guided sextant biopsies of the prostate for the detection of prostate cancer. *J Urol.* 1998 Feb;159(2):471–5; discussion 475–6.

2. Loeb S, Vellekoop A, Ahmed HU, Catto J, et al. Systematic review of complications of prostate biopsy. *European Urology.* 2013; Accepted 24 May 2013, Published online 4 June 2013.

3. Klein T, Palisaar RJ, Holz A, Brock M, Noldus J, Hinkel A. The impact of prostate biopsy and periprostatic nerve block on erectile and voiding function: a prospective study. *J Urol.* 2010 Oct; 184(4):1447–52.

4. Hoeks CM, Barentsz JO, Hambrock T, et al. Prostate cancer: multiparametric MR imaging for detection, localization, and staging. *Radiology.* 2011 Oct;261(1):46–66.

5. NYU Langone Medical Center and the Sperling Prostate Cancer Center.

6. Yerram NK, Volkin D, Turkbey B, et al. Low suspicion lesions on multiparametric magnetic resonance imaging predict for the absence of high-risk prostate cancer. *BJU Int.* 2012 Dec;110(11 Pt B):E783–8.

7. Arumainayagam N, Ahmed HU, Moore CM, et al. Multiparametric MR Imaging for detection of clinically significant prostate cancer: a validation cohort study with transperineal template prostate mapping as the reference standard. *Radiology.* 2013 Apr 5.

8. Numao N, Yoshida S, Komai Y, et al. Usefulness of prebiopsy multi-parametric magnetic resonance imaging and clinical variables to reduce initial prostate biopsy in men with suspected clinically localized prostate cancer. *J Urol.* 2013 Mar 6.

9. Noguchi M, Stamey TA, McNeal JE, Yemoto CM. Relationship between systematic biopsies and histological features of 222 radical prostatectomy specimens: lack of prediction of tumor significance for men with nonpalpable prostate cancer. *J Urol.* 2001 Jul;166(1): 104–9; discussion 109–10.

10. D'Amico AV, Whittington R, Malkowicz SB, et al. Biochemical outcome after radical prostatectomy, external beam radiation therapy, or interstitial radiation therapy for clinically localized prostate cancer. *JAMA* 1998; 280:969–974; and Greene FL. American Joint Committee on Cancer. American Cancer Society. *AJCC Cancer Staging Manual*. 6th Ed. New York, NY: Springer-Verlag; 2002.
11. Edge, Stephen B. et al. eds. *AJCC Cancer Staging Manual*, 7th edition. Springer. 2010.

Patient Checklist

Bring this checklist with you to your next doctor's visit to get the answers you need to stay healthy.

☐ Why are you recommending a biopsy for me? _____
_____
_____
_____

☐ What imaging technique do you recommend for my biopsy and why?
_____
_____
_____

☐ Is multiparametric MRI an option for me? _____
_____
_____
_____

☐ If my first biopsy is negative, what is your suggested follow-up and why? _____
_____
_____
_____

☐ What is the risk of my cancer spreading based on my biopsy pathology report? _____
_____
_____
_____

☐ Will I need to take antibiotics before and/or after my procedure to minimize the chance of serious infection? _____
_____
_____
_____

Visit www.sprypubprostate.com to download a printable checklist.

CHAPTER FIVE

I Have Prostate Cancer: Now What?

Two Men, Different Stories

Sean is a 52-year-old architect who was recently remarried and is visiting his doctor for a routine physical. The doctor notices a questionable hardness during his prostate exam. His PSA test is slightly elevated at 4.2 ng/mL. His doctor orders an mpMRI, which detects a small (8 mm region of interest) area of abnormality in the prostate that is suspicious for cancer. And a follow-up prostate biopsy confirms the diagnosis of a slow-growing prostate cancer.

In discussing treatment options, Sean expresses his great concern about the possibility of loss of sexual or bladder function with surgery. His doctor explains that his cancer is confined to the prostate capsule and likely extremely slow growing. Due to his young age, he is not an ideal candidate for treating it with "active surveillance," a management strategy that forgoes surgery or radiation treatment for a protocol of careful follow-up and regular testing. Sean isn't sure if he likes the idea of letting cancer grow in his prostate and tells his doctor he needs time to consider his options.

Jim is a 68-year-old retiree who is recovering from a recent heart attack ten months ago and is doing well. He visits his doctor because he is having trouble with excessive urination, especially at night.

Normally, Jim tries to avoid the doctor's office whenever he can get away with it, but his wife is worried. So he agreed to a checkup. His PSA is found to be at 4.8 ng/mL; up from his last PSA about three years ago, which was 1.8 ng/mL. His doctor repeated the PSA to make sure there was no laboratory error, and the second test result is 4.9 ng/mL. On digital rectal exam he had a slightly tender prostate. He was given a course of antibiotics, and a second test a month later is 4.9 ng/mL. An MRI shows a single 15 mm × 10 mm highly suspicious region of interest, and a targeted 3-D co-registered biopsy detects a Gleason 6 prostate cancer. The random biopsies are negative.

Jim's doctor also explains the option of active surveillance. Other than the mild urination problems, Jim has no symptoms. He is worried that prostate surgery may take a further toll on his heart. If the cancer is not spreading or growing quickly, he thinks he would rather leave it alone than spend even more of his retirement years visiting doctors. He tells his doctor he'll discuss it with his wife.

The Patient-Doctor Partnership

Ultimately, you are responsible for your own healthcare. Your doctor is, of course, an important part of figuring out health problems and helping you treat them, but when it comes to decision making and following through on treatment and care, the buck stops with you.

A diagnosis of cancer is overwhelming, and it can be tempting to sit back in shock and let your doctor take control. But this is where your partnership is even more critical. Finding the "right" treatment for your prostate cancer isn't about looking at cancer cells under a microscope and then applying a treatment algorithm. It's about looking at you as a whole person—your family, job, likes/dislikes, habits, personality, culture—and then finding the treatment that will work best to maintain both your health and happiness.

Talking to Your Doctor

Full disclosure and open communication are important when working with your doctor to treat your prostate cancer. That means frank discussion about sexual performance and habits, emotional well-being, and other potentially sensitive topics. Remember that the patient-doctor relationship is highly confidential and having these conversations will lead to better care for you.

In an ideal world, we'd spend at least 45 minutes with each patient, do a thorough history and evaluation, and have time left over to talk about the big game Sunday. This is the kind of patient care we all envisioned when we were in medical school. Unfortunately, scheduling and emergencies make these types of visits a rarity, and 9 times out of 10 we need to get right to the business at hand when we walk into the exam room.

We ask you to understand this unavoidable hazard of the profession and help us minimize any impact to you by being prepared. If you were given forms to fill out prior to the visit, make sure they are complete when you arrive. Write a list of questions you have before the appointment and bring it along, with a pen to take notes. Sometimes it's a good idea to bring a spouse or significant other as a second set of ears.

A Treatment Team

While a urologist typically diagnoses prostate cancer, your treatment may involve a number of other specialists, including a radiation oncologist, an interventional radiologist, and others. All the physicians involved with your prostate cancer care can and should coordinate treatment and records among themselves.

If you have other chronic health conditions for which you are being treated, it's important to let your urologist know about these. Likewise, you should make sure your other doctors are aware that you are being treated for prostate cancer. Sometimes, treatment and medicines for one health condition can interact with those for another, so sharing your cancer care and health information is important.

While electronic health records will eventually make this kind of information sharing easier, it's still up to you, the patient, to ensure that all of your doctors are on the same page. Sometimes this can seem like a monumental task, particularly if you have a complicated health history. Here are some practical tips to make it easier:

- **Keep a written record of all the medications you take.** This should include dosage and special instructions. List over-the-counter medicines and supplements, as well. Bring this list to all of your doctor's appointments.
- **Sign release forms.** As you visit all of your regular physicians, ask for release forms to allow them to share needed health information with each other. You may have to update these annually depending on the office policy.
- **Always request a hard copy of laboratory and pathology results.** If your healthcare providers have trouble sharing information in a timely manner, you will have a copy on hand to provide to another office.

What kind of doctor should treat my prostate cancer?

Although you may see urologists, radiation oncologists, internists, and other doctors during prostate cancer treatment, a urologist usually heads up your prostate cancer treatment team. A urologist has had specialized treatment in diseases of the male urinary and reproductive tract and is most familiar with diseases of the prostate.

Second Opinions

It's important that you are confident in your prostate cancer treatment decision. If you're uncomfortable or still have questions after you've had a full consultation with a doctor, you need to get a second opinion for your own peace of mind. Realize that it's possible that the second opinion may be different than the first, which might trigger the need to seek a third opinion. At the end of the day, you need to be at peace with the decision you make.

Because different specialists focus on different types of prostate cancer treatment, it is helpful to visit different doctors to learn more about your options when you are not sure which path to take. For example, a urologic surgeon can offer the most insight into prostate surgery, a radiation oncologist can tell you all about radiation therapy, and an interventional radiologist can explain MRI and prostate ablation. Each of these specialists is very comfortable and confident in their own treatment protocol. The best case scenario is to find a practice or prostate cancer center such as the Smilow Comprehensive Prostate Cancer Center where these different specialists work collaboratively with one another to provide you with integrated care.

My doctor is recommending that I get my prostate removed, but I'm not sure. Is it wrong to ask him about getting a second opinion?

Don't be afraid of offending your doctor by seeking a second opinion. Second opinions are quite common in cancer treatment. Physicians understand that you are the one ultimately responsible for your own health and well-being, and that gathering as much information as possible is part of being an informed patient. Most doctors are happy to provide a referral; if not, ask your health insurance company or check with the American Urological Association for a urologist in your area.

You should also realize that there's nothing wrong with not getting a second opinion if you are comfortable with the first one. Many patients say, "You know, I saw this doctor, he communicated very clearly with me. I'm very confident with what he said to me, and I don't need another opinion." And that's fine, too.

The "Art" of Prostate Cancer Treatment

Prostate cancer is unique in that there is almost as much "art" to appropriate diagnosis and treatment as there is science. The science tells us what types of cancers are more likely to be aggressive and what percentage of men may benefit from a certain kind of treatment.

But it doesn't give us the full picture of what the right choice is for you as an individual. And as doctors, we have a responsibility to each patient, not to population statistics.

From screening to treatment, one size certainly does not fit all in prostate cancer. Every cancer is biologically different, and every patient has different personal needs for treatment based on health, age, lifestyle, and emotional needs. Looking at all of these factors is the best way to determine what is "right" for you.

Finding Your Treatment Path

Treatment for prostate cancer runs the gamut from surgical removal to a "wait, watch, and see" approach of scheduled screening and careful observation known as *active surveillance*. Newer innovative methods of treatment use MRI to target the cancerous tissue and destroy it with lasers (described in detail in chapter 8).

With early-stage cancers that are confined to the prostate, patients have four major options for treatment: (1) surgical removal of the prostate gland (radical prostatectomy), (2) radiation therapy to the prostate gland, (3) partial or whole gland ablation, and (4) active surveillance. You may be a candidate for more than one of these. To help determine the best treatment path for you as an individual, you and your doctor should consider the following:

- **Age**—A 50-year-old man usually has very different personal and health needs than an 80-year-old man. For men in the very late years of life, surgery or other invasive treatments for prostate cancer will do little to prolong their lives and can cause significant harm.
- **Health Status**—If you have other serious health conditions, they are a consideration in your prostate cancer treatment. Your doctor should explain how your overall health will be influenced by various treatment choices. For example, men with preexisting bowel diseases such as ulcerative colitis, diverticulitis, or Crohn's disease would be poor candidates for radiation therapy.

- **Psychological Impact**—Your emotional well-being is just as important as your physical health. Some men find it difficult to cope with a treatment path where cancer is left in the prostate and monitored (active surveillance). Others may have extreme anxiety and depression around the idea of sexual or urinary side effects from surgery. Minimizing stress around prostate cancer treatment is an important part of overall patient health.
- **Individual Needs and Lifestyle**—Jobs, family dynamics, finances, sexual activity, personal passions—all of these are a consideration in choosing an appropriate prostate cancer treatment. As your doctor discusses the side effects and outcomes of different treatments, think about how they will affect the way you actually live your life.

In an ideal world, your doctor would discuss all of these factors with you in detail to help guide your treatment choice. But with the time and scheduling pressures of the typical doctor's office visit, things can get overlooked. Bring the patient checklist at the end of this chapter to your doctor's office when discussing treatment options. And remember, in the vast majority of cases, there is no rush to come to a decision as you sit in your doctor's office hearing your options. If you need time to contemplate your choices and discuss them with family, take it.

What is the best treatment for me and my cancer?

The best treatment is one that will prolong your life without damaging your overall quality of life. This will be different for every man based on his personal circumstances and the specific characteristics of the prostate cancer itself. A full and frank discussion with your doctor is the best way to determine what course of treatment is right for you.

Living with Prostate Cancer: Active Surveillance

Active surveillance is a treatment option for men with slow-growing prostate cancer that is not causing symptoms, is confined to the prostate gland, and is at low risk for metastasizing, or spreading. Men with a Gleason score of 6 are the ideal candidates for active surveillance.

With treatments such as surgery, ablation, and radiation, once the procedure is done there isn't much required of you, the patient, other than routine follow-up PSA levels. But active surveillance is a bit different. The emphasis is on "active" and requires full cooperation and commitment to careful follow-up and monitoring, and a patient who is capable and willing to cooperate with this treatment plan.

What Is Active Surveillance?

First of all, let's talk about what active surveillance is not. It is not "doing nothing" about your prostate cancer. It is a choice to carefully monitor your cancer with a schedule of PSA tests, DREs, imaging, and biopsies. Your doctor will recommend a screening schedule based on your cancer profile. If at any point your prostate cancer shows signs of progression, then a more aggressive treatment (e.g., surgery or radiation) can be started. The importance of surveillance cannot be over-emphasized. Dr. Lepor has published data showing that between 50% and 70% of men deemed candidates for active surveillance harbor more intermediate- or high-risk disease.[1] The expectation is that surveillance will identify these individuals at a later time while the disease is curable and no harm is done by deferring treatment.

I have cancer ... and you think I should watch it grow?

Active surveillance is not simply "watching cancer grow." It is a careful monitoring system designed to maintain a man's health and quality of life. And it is only recommended for men who have very low-risk cancers confined to the prostate gland that are not causing symptoms (an estimated 70% of men diagnosed with prostate cancer). Of these, over 90% will elect to have surgery or radiation treatment for prostate cancer. And the majority of men will experience at least one negative side effect from that treatment.[2] The goal of active surveillance is to not over-treat men who don't need it, while still catching any progression in their cancer at a treatable stage.

Pros and Cons

Men who decide on active surveillance do not have to face the immediate side effects or potential complications of other more invasive treatments. This often makes it a good choice for older men or men with other serious health conditions for whom surgery might be too dangerous. It may also be an option for younger or healthier men with extremely slow-growing cancers who do not want to deal with the complications of more aggressive treatments at this stage in their lives.

However, it can be difficult for many men to live with the idea that they have prostate cancer. With surgery, once the procedure is over, you have the peace of mind of knowing that your cancer is likely gone. With active surveillance, you need to be comfortable with the fact that you are living with cancer, presumably one that is slow growing and currently not life threatening.

The major risk associated with active surveillance is the possibility that the cancer will spread beyond your prostate gland while on active surveillance. However, the schedule of monitoring your doctor recommends is designed to catch any significant growth at its earliest stage.

For a doctor, active surveillance can be a difficult choice to offer. It's a relatively new idea, especially when it comes to cancer. When certain conditions are borderline or mild, such as cholesterol or blood pressure, a "let's wait and see" approach is something with which we can deal. But in general, we are trained to be definitive in our approach to cancers. And when we're talking about cancer, an invasive disease that can kill, the wait and see approach is a difficult one to adjust to. As more long-term research about the benefits of active surveillance in certain men is published, physicians will likely become more comfortable with the idea. The majority of data suggests that active surveillance is a safe option for appropriately selected men who comply with the surveillance regimen.

Is It Right for You?

Ultimately, it is your decision about whether or not active surveillance is right for you. If your doctor recommends active surveillance, ask him to clearly explain what your schedule of monitoring will be. Some doctors may refer to active surveillance as *watchful waiting* or *expectant management*. Remember that active surveillance is a relatively new option in prostate cancer treatment; if your doctor mentions any of these terms, make sure he tells you exactly what he means by them.

Part of the active surveillance decision is being comfortable with the schedule of follow-up screening. If you aren't sure you will be able to commit to regular screening appointments, you might want to consider a different course of treatment.

Putting It All Together

Let's return to Sean and Jim, our two patients considering active surveillance. After talking to his wife and doing some research on the Internet, Sean decides to pursue active surveillance. He feels great and the thought of losing sexual function or bladder control with surgery, even temporarily, is highly concerning to him. He and his doctor set up a PSA and DRE screening in three months, a repeat MRI in six months, and a repeat biopsy in a year. One year later, the PSA, MRI, and DRE are stable, and the repeat biopsy shows a Gleason 6 cancer. Sean's cancer continues to be low risk and he remains on active surveillance.

Jim also opts for active surveillance. He was worried about undergoing any kind of surgical procedure in light of his recent heart attack. Despite his dislike of doctors' offices, he and his wife agree that regular follow-up is better for his overall health than surgery or radiation right now. His doctor sets a schedule of three month PSA and DRE, and a repeat MRI and biopsy in one year.

Over the one year, Jim's PSA progressively rises to a level of 6.2. The MRI shows modest growth of the region of interest, and a repeat biopsy shows a Gleason 7 cancer. Jim's doctor explains that he has been up-staged to a medium-risk cancer that is growing based on his rising PSA and MRI. At this point, Jim elects to undergo an MRI-guided laser ablation under local anesthesia as an outpatient. He realizes that there will be uncertainties as to whether the cancer will be totally eradicated, and he will require a modified active surveillance protocol. Jim goes back to work two days after the ablation and doesn't have any complications of the procedure. A repeat biopsy six months later shows no residual cancer. So far, so good.

References

1. Mufarrij P, Sankin A, Godoy G, Lepor H. Pathologic outcomes of candidates for active surveillance undergoing radical prostatectomy. *Urology*. 2010 Sep;76(3):689–92. doi: 10.1016/j.urology.2009.12.075.

2. Hayes JH, Ollendorf DA, Pearson SD, et al. Active surveillance compared with initial treatment for men with low-risk prostate cancer: a decision analysis. *JAMA*. 2010 Dec 1;304(21):2373–80.

Patient Checklist

Bring this checklist with you to your next doctor's visit to get the answers you need to stay healthy.

☐ What treatment(s) are appropriate for my particular kind of prostate cancer? _____

_____

_____

_____

☐ Do any of my existing health conditions make successful treatment more difficult? _____

_____

_____

_____

☐ What are the potential side effects of the treatment(s) you propose?

_____

_____

_____

☐ Am I a candidate for active surveillance? Why or why not? _____

_____

_____

_____

☐ If active surveillance is an option for me, what is your recommended screening schedule? _____

_____

_____

_____

Visit www.sprypubprostate.com to download a printable checklist.

CHAPTER SIX

Treatment Choices: Removing the Prostate

One Man's Story

John is a 68-year-old man with a family history of prostate cancer. John's father, Bill, was diagnosed with the disease at age 65. At the time, PSA testing was not available. Bill was having problems with urinary frequency and stream, so he visited the urologist, who felt a suspicious lump during DRE. Further tests revealed a tumor. Bill underwent radiation therapy. Three years later, he complained of back pain, and a bone scan revealed cancer throughout his spine. He underwent a bilateral orchiectomy (removal of the testes) and his bone pain miraculously resolved. Unfortunately, the cancer recurred three years later and he died at age 72. John vividly remembers the misery his father experienced the last few years of life with bone pain and ultimately liver failure.

Due to his family history, John started annual PSA testing at age 40. His PSA level was consistently less than 2.5 ng/mL until 3 years ago, when it rose slightly to 2.7 ng/mL. The PSA results the following 2 years were 3.4 and 4.0 ng/mL. This steady and significant rise prompted his doctor to send John to a urologist, who ordered a biopsy. The biopsy found a Gleason 6 cancer confined to the left lobe of the prostate.

John's urologist discussed three options with him for his low-risk cancer: active surveillance, radiation therapy, or radical prostatectomy (surgery to remove the prostate). He explained that John's cancer may not be life threatening and that while surgery and radiation would likely cure the cancer, they did carry some risk and side effects. John listened carefully, but from an emotional perspective, he had made up his mind. He had witnessed firsthand what it was like to die of cancer. He felt strongly that surgery to remove the prostate and the cancer within it was the best choice for him.

An Early History of Prostate Removal Surgery

The first radical prostatectomy (RP) surgeries took place in the early 1900s. At this time, there were no good prostate cancer screening tools available, and when men were diagnosed, they usually had advanced disease. With these early surgeries, the prostate was removed through an incision between the scrotum and anus (the perineum). Most men were not cured, and the mortality rate was high due to the lack of antibiotics and poor anesthesia technique. Many were incontinent and almost all ended up impotent.

In the late 1940s, a new surgical technique for radical prostatectomy, known as the retropubic approach, gained popularity. This involved removing the prostate through an incision in the lower abdomen. The primary advantage of the retropubic approach over the perineal approach was the ability to remove the lymph nodes through the same incision and test them for the presence of cancer. Because most men at this time still had advanced disease (again, before the advent of PSA as a screening tool), this was considered an advantage. If the lymph nodes were positive, the surgery was often aborted. The major disadvantage of the retropubic approach was greater bleeding, often resulting in multiple blood transfusions.[1]

Today, surgical advances in both radical retropubic prostatectomy (RRP) and radical perineal prostatectomy (RPP) (see figure 10) have made these surgeries much more effective while cutting the risk of bleeding, nerve damage, and other common complications.

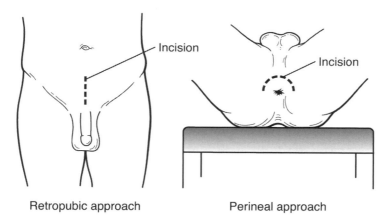

Retropubic approach   Perineal approach

Figure 10. Retropubic and perineal approaches to radical prostatectomy surgery.

Why can't they just cut out only the cancer from my prostate?

A major justification for radical or total removal of the prostate gland is that prostate cancer is typically *multifocal*. This means that it is usually found in several different regions of the prostate rather than just one small region of the gland. But as discussed elsewhere in this book, the random systematic biopsy most men get is notoriously unreliable for determining the site, extent, and aggressiveness of prostate cancer within the gland. Therefore, the most reliable way to ensure that all cancer is taken out is to surgically remove the entire prostate.

As imaging (mpMRI) and targeted biopsies become more reliable, new molecular markers of aggressive disease are developed, and targeted ablation becomes more widely available, men may instead choose to undergo less invasive ablation treatment. This treatment is described in detail in chapter 8.

Nerve-Sparing RP: A Surgical Revolution

The greatest advance in radical prostatectomy was the anatomic nerve-sparing radical retropubic prostatectomy. Before the 1980s, one of the major complications of RP was that virtually all men were left impotent by the surgery. In 1985, Dr. Lepor was the first to show the precise pathway for the microscopic nerves that control erectile function. These microscopic nerves responsible for erections are located very close to the prostate. These tiny nerves were inadvertently damaged during traditional RP surgery.[2]

In the 1980s, Dr. Patrick Walsh developed a surgical technique to preserve these erection nerves during RP surgery in selected men with prostate cancer clinically localized to the gland.[3] Potency rates rose dramatically with the use of nerve-sparing radical prostatectomy.[4] Some studies show potency rates as high as 86% eighteen months after surgery.[5]

It's important for men to realize that regardless of what type of surgery they have, at best their potency level will only return to the level it was prior to treatment. In other words, it is unrealistic to expect your erections to be better than they were. Your doctor may have you complete an assessment known as the International Index of Erectile Function (IIEF) to establish your levels of erectile function and sexual satisfaction prior to treatment.[6]

Another advantage of the nerve-sparing RP approach is that it incorporates surgical methods to control bleeding from the dorsal venous complex, the group of blood vessels that run alongside the penis, prostate, and bladder. These surgical methods greatly reduced blood loss and also made it easier for a surgeon to better see the prostate and other important anatomic landmarks (see figure 11).

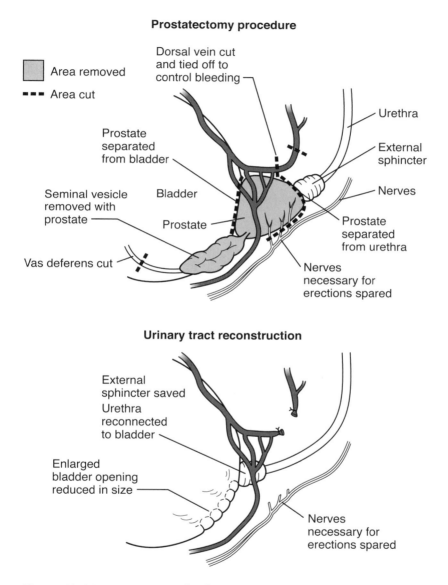

Prostatectomy procedure

Dorsal vein cut and tied off to control bleeding

Area removed

Area cut

Prostate separated from bladder

Seminal vesicle removed with prostate

Vas deferens cut

Bladder

Prostate

Urethra

External sphincter

Nerves

Prostate separated from urethra

Nerves necessary for erections spared

Urinary tract reconstruction

External sphincter saved

Urethra reconnected to bladder

Enlarged bladder opening reduced in size

Nerves necessary for erections spared

Figure 11. Nerve-sparing radical prostatectomy. The surgeon rebuilds the urinary tract, pulling the bladder down to bridge the space connecting the urethra and urethral sphincter.

Am I a candidate for nerve-sparing surgery?

Men with localized prostate cancer confined to the gland may be eligible for nerve-sparing surgery. If your cancer has penetrated the capsule, or outer surface, of the prostate gland, this type of surgery is not appropriate.

If perineural invasion is seen in the prostate biopsy, you may not be a good candidate for nerve-sparing surgery. Perineural invasion means that cancer has penetrated the nerves of the prostate and may potentially invade outside the prostatic capsule. Other factors your surgeon may consider in whether or not to offer nerve-sparing surgery include your Gleason score and tumor volume.[7]

Robotic-Assisted RP: Superior or Marketing Ploy?

Robotic-assisted laparoscopic radical prostatectomy (RALRP) began in the early 2000s. In RALRP, several small incisions are made in the abdomen, and the surgery is performed through these openings using small cameras and robotic assistance. The robotic approach was popularized primarily by direct-to-consumer marketing as a "minimally invasive" approach to RP.[8] Today, approximately 70% of RPs are performed with robotic assistance.

Comparative effectiveness data fail to show any meaningful advantage of robotic over the traditional open approach as far as technical complications, oncological control, continence, potency, or patient satisfaction.[9] In fact, some comparative effectiveness studies suggest that the robotic approach is inferior to the open approach.[10] Consider the evidence:

- **Positive Surgical Margins**—A publication from Brigham and Women's Hospital, an affiliated and world-renowned hospital of Harvard Medical School, found that robotic prostatectomy was 1.9 times more likely to produce positive surgical margins than an open RP procedure.[11] A positive margin means that the pathologist has found cancer cells on the edge of the removed surgical specimen indicating cancer may have been left behind.

- **Incontinence and Potency**—A study of Medicare patients found that robotic-assisted RP was associated with worse urinary incontinence than open radical prostatectomy, and potency across the two procedures was equivalent.[12]
- **Patient Satisfaction**—A publication from Duke Medical Center reported that men undergoing robotic-assisted RP are more likely to be dissatisfied with their outcome compared to the open RP.[13]
- **Pain and Length of Hospital Stay**—A publication from Vanderbilt Hospital reported that pain and length of hospital stay were no different between robotic-assisted and open RP.[14]

Given the evidence, we feel there is no justification for the increased cost of robotic prostatectomy and the consequences associated with its learning curve. Dr. Lepor has published extensively on this topic. If you are considering surgery, we encourage you to visit the Smilow Comprehensive Prostate Cancer Center website at prostate-cancer.med.nyu.edu to read the latest news and research on robotic-assisted and open prostatectomy.

It's important for men to understand that with any surgical treatment the level of experience of the surgeon is critical. As with just about any task, the more you perform it, the more skill you gain. Whatever surgery you are considering, be sure to ask your urologist how many procedures he has performed and what overall success rates he can share regarding his specific outcomes.

Is there any advantage to robotic-assisted radical prostatectomy?

The only advantage of the robotic-assisted RP over the open approach is less bleeding during the operation. However, men who undergo an open RP surgery may be given injections of erythropoietin (a drug that increases red blood cell production) before surgery. This practice has been proven to decrease the need for postsurgical blood transfusions.[15]

What Are the Potential Complications of RP?

Possible complications from both open and robotic-assisted RP are unintended injury to the bowel and major nerves or blood vessels. Fortunately, in the hands of expert surgeons skilled in RP, these injuries are very uncommon. Recently, there have been reports in the media that severe injuries and even postoperative mortalities have been attributed to inexperienced and inadequately trained robotic-assisted surgeons.[16,17]

Immediate postoperative complications may include bleeding, which will often become evident in the first few hours following surgery. For men undergoing RP who have preexisting heart disease, cardiac enzymes are drawn after surgery to ensure there has not been a "silent" heart attack.

One potentially fatal postoperative complication is a pulmonary embolus, a blood clot blocking an artery in the lungs. This happens when blood clots form in the pelvis or lower extremities during or after surgery and travel up to the lungs. Any ankle swelling or pain in the calf muscles following surgery should be reported to your doctor immediately. Shortness of breath or chest pain while breathing is a sign that a blood clot may be in the lungs. This is a medical emergency and you should get medical attention immediately if this happens to you.

Radical prostatectomy involves removing the prostate and suturing the bladder to the urethra. In a small number (<5%) of cases, scar tissue may develop at this site, which creates a stricture (or narrowing) of the urethra. If this happens, it usually occurs within the first 3 months after surgery. Men will experience a slowing of the urine stream and at times worsening of incontinence. These men may need a simple outpatient procedure that dilates, or stretches, the scar tissue to open the urethra back up. In rare cases, strictures will recur and require additional surgical interventions.

Other more common complications from radical prostatectomy surgery that may persist for many months include erectile dysfunction

(ED), lower urinary tract symptoms (LUTS), and urinary incontinence. Fortunately, these typically improve over time, and there are treatments available if they do not.

Is there any treatment or preparation required before surgery?

Before RP surgery, men will undergo routine preoperative testing including blood tests, electrocardiogram (ECG), and a chest X-ray. Men with heart disease may also need a stress test and should also make sure their primary care physician and/or cardiologist are aware of the upcoming surgery. All men should stop taking aspirin-containing products, nonsteroidal anti-inflammatory agents, and omega-3 supplements one week before RP. An enema is given the night before and morning of surgery. You should also not drink or eat after midnight the night before surgery.

Some surgeons recommend that patients bank their own blood before surgery in case a transfusion is required. Others, including Dr. Lepor, do not recommend this approach, as less than 5% of men undergoing RP will require blood transfusion, and the procedure makes men anemic.

What to Expect after Surgery

Your postsurgical instructions may vary depending upon your specific surgical procedure, your health history, and your surgeon. Dr. Lepor recommends that his RP patients do not do any heavy lifting or driving immediately following surgery. Men may resume heavy lifting in two weeks and may drive as soon as they are off of narcotics for pain control. Other than these minor restrictions, men are generally free to resume normal activity. They may shower, have a drink with dinner, enjoy an unrestricted diet, be a passenger in the car, take a walk, and climb upstairs the day of discharge, which is typically after only one night in the hospital.

You will leave the hospital with a urinary catheter still in place, which is inserted into the penis during your surgery. The catheter usually stays in about a week while the connection between the bladder and urethra heals; your doctor will remove it at a follow-up visit.

Within 2 weeks, 50% of men will have returned to work after open RP. Within a month, 50% will resume unrestricted physical activities.[18] That means if you run marathons, you can get back on the road in four weeks. How quickly you return to work and exercise is influenced by your blood count at discharge and how quickly your catheter is removed following surgery.

Urinary Control

Urinary incontinence is the involuntary loss of urine and is one of the biggest fears of men undergoing RP. Most men will experience some level of temporary urinary incontinence and will need to wear protective pads. With an experienced surgeon, permanent incontinence is extremely unlikely, and most men regain what they consider a socially acceptable level of bladder control within months following surgery. In Dr. Lepor's practice, he reports continence rates of 80%, 90%, 93%, and 97% at 3, 6, 12, and 24 months, respectively, after open RP.

It is important to realize that for some men, continence does not mean perfect urinary control, which is defined as never leaking a drop. In fact, 24.5% of adult U.S. men report experiencing occasional leakage with strenuous exercise, a vigorous cough, or when bending down to pick something up (known as *stress incontinence*).[19] In most cases, they will wear no pad or a tiny protective pad. Men with an occasional leakage prior to or after RP consider themselves continent since it causes no impairment of daily or quality of life.

I'm still experiencing significant incontinence and my surgery was a month ago. Is there any treatment that can help?

You can try Kegel exercises. This involves contracting the pelvic floor muscles to strengthen them. It's an exercise that is easy to do and can be performed anytime and anywhere. Just tighten the muscles you use to stop your urine stream, hold for 3 seconds, and release for 3 seconds. Repeat 10 to 15 times a session, and do these sessions as many times as you are comfortable doing each day. A biofeedback program may also be helpful. This involves seeing a biofeedback therapist to relearn how to relax your bladder and tighten your pelvic floor muscles using instruments that measure electrical activity in these muscles.

Fortunately, virtually all men regain their continence after RP. For the small minority who do not, there are surgical procedures that will greatly improve or totally resolve the incontinence. For minor persistent incontinence, a male sling procedure that elevates the bladder neck with a synthetic mesh "sling" has excellent outcomes. When persistent incontinence is severe, an artificial urinary sphincter can be implanted. This device is a small inflatable cuff that surrounds the urethra. An inflation bulb is connected to it, which is placed in the scrotum. The cuff can be inflated and deflated at will to allow urination. However, this is a more involved surgery, and the device may need replacement after ten years. Therefore, it is usually not recommended unless all other options to regain continence have failed.

Other lower urinary tract symptoms may also occur besides incontinence. These include storage symptoms (urinary frequency and urgency, getting up at night repeatedly to urinate) and emptying symptoms (decrease force of stream, sensation of incomplete urinary stream, interrupted urinary stream, dribbling). Even without RP surgery, LUTS are common in the aging male population, as the prostate often enlarges with age and affects urine flow. A survey of more than 5,000 U.S. men age 65 and older found that 46% experience moderate to severe LUTS.[20] Interestingly, the majority of men who experience LUTS before prostate cancer diagnosis and who undergo RP will experience relief from these LUTS after surgery.[21]

Is any one type of surgery better for improving my chances of not losing erectile function?

As described earlier in this chapter, nerve-sparing radical prostatectomy is currently the best available option for men who are worried about impotency after surgery. When performed by a skilled surgeon who is experienced in nerve-sparing RP, your chances of regaining erectile function after surgery are excellent. If your prostate cancer is confined to the prostate gland, you may be a candidate for this type of surgery.

Radical Prostatectomy and Sexual Function

Most men who have RP will experience erectile dysfunction. Recovering the ability to have an erection after RP often takes up to two years, although men can still continue to recover up to five years after RP. In some cases, ED is permanent. How quickly ED resolves depends on several factors, including age, the experience of the surgeon, erectile function before surgery, the type of RP performed, and whether or not the patient has existing heart disease. For men under 70 with no risk factors who have bilateral nerve-sparing RP, about 71% will regain erections adequate for intercourse with or without the use of a PDE-5 inhibitor drug such as Viagra, Cialis, or Levitra.[22]

New York University Langone Medical Center (NYULMC) was one of the centers that participated in a controlled randomized study examining whether 50 mg a day of Viagra was superior to a placebo at resolving ED. Men who took Viagra for nine months were more likely to experience normal erections at one year than those on placebo.[23] Based on this and other studies, most urologists will recommend a daily or every other day PDE-5 inhibitor drug.

These studies have also led to the concept of penile rehabilitation in RP patients. At NYULMC, men who are eager and motivated to regain erections are started on PDE-5 inhibitors immediately following RP. By three months, most have regained continence. Men are encouraged to start penile injections twice a week and resume having sexual intercourse. Alternatively, men can use a penile vacuum device (figure 12) to achieve a rigid penis for intercourse. This approach allows many couples to resume intercourse while awaiting the natural return of erectile function.

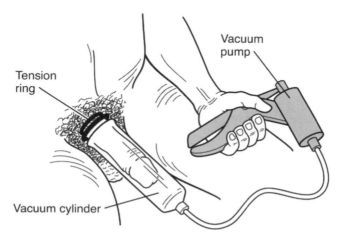

Figure 12. A penile vacuum device may be used to achieve a rigid penis for intercourse. The vacuum device consists of a clear plastic cylinder with an aperture at one end that is placed over the penile shaft. At the other end of the cylinder is a pump mechanism that is used to generate negative pressure within the cylinder. There are a number of medical equipment companies that have specially designed devices that are carefully constructed so that a limited amount of pressure is allowed to develop, reducing the likelihood of pressure-induced penile injury. Only FDA-approved devices should be used.

If my erectile function doesn't return, do I have any options to restore it?

Of course, many men will experience pleasurable orgasms even without an erection. An erection is required for penetration only, and many couples still enjoy intimacy without intercourse. However, you do have options if ED is an issue for you and medication isn't helping. At any time penile injections (intracavernous injections) may be started. These injections cause the blood vessels in the penis to dilate, allowing blood flow and erection. For men who experienced good erections before surgery, injections will almost always be effective. However, they may not be effective in men with atherosclerotic disease who have blockages to the arteries that feed the penis. If penile injections are ineffective, a penile prosthesis may be surgically implanted that uses a fluid pump and inflatable cylinder to achieve an erection.

ED is just one way that prostate cancer surgery impacts overall sexual function. Dwindling libido, less pleasurable orgasms, and pain during orgasm are also potential problems. There is also the possibility of incontinence occurring during foreplay or orgasm, which can be disconcerting and embarrassing to many men.

It's important to note that RP eliminates the capability to produce semen in all men. For most older men and couples this is not an issue. But for younger men and couples currently contemplating having children, sperm banking before RP is recommended.

Can My Cancer Return?

The overwhelming majority of men are diagnosed with low- or intermediate-risk disease that has not metastasized to lymph nodes, the skeletal system, or other organs like the liver or lungs. For these men, surgery to remove the prostate is essentially a cure for prostate cancer.

Men with high-risk disease have a greater likelihood of having metastasis. Imaging studies such as a bone scan or abdominal/pelvic CT or MRI should be performed in these men. It is possible for imaging studies to be falsely negative when metastases are too small to detect.

The goal of RP is to remove the entire prostate along with the cancer. Because the prostate is the source of PSA, we expect PSA tests after the surgery to be undetectable. But any residual prostate or prostate cancer will raise the PSA level after surgery. In properly performed RP, benign prostate tissue will raise the PSA in less than 1% of cases. And if the PSA is due to benign prostate tissue, then the rate of PSA change will be very slow.

If cancer returns, the PSA will be detectable years before the disease shows up on imaging tests or causes symptoms. There is a consensus that a biochemical recurrence (BCR) of prostate cancer after prostatectomy is defined by a PSA > 0.2 ng/mL measured on at least two occasions. BCR indicates that PSA is rising and cancer is returning. Imaging studies at the time of BCR are typically negative since the tumor is microscopic at this time. One of the best ways to differentiate whether the recurrence is local or systemic is the time to recurrence and the PSA doubling time (PSADT). PSADT is a calculation of the time it takes for a man's PSA to double in value and is an indicator of the aggressiveness of a prostate cancer.

My cancer has returned after surgery. Should I have radiation?

There are some urologists and radiation oncologists who will recommend adjuvant radiation therapy (ART) if there are high-risk factors for biochemical recurrence. This is termed *adjuvant RT* since there is no hard evidence that residual disease is present. The term adjuvant indicates a treatment that enhances or assists another primary treatment. It is essentially a backup therapy.

We disagree with this approach since this will subject between 50% and 60% of men to unnecessary radiation therapy along with its side effects. Instead, we recommend salvage RT or delivery of RT only when there is evidence of a BCR. The decision to offer salvage RT should be determined by the rate of change of PSA, the time to BCR, Gleason score, and evidence of positive margins. Chapter 7 has more information on radiation therapy.

Putting It All Together

John underwent an open nerve-sparing radical retropubic prosta-tectomy. His postsurgical biopsy report showed a Gleason 7 cancer that had penetrated the prostate capsule but had not yet spread any further. The surgical margins were negative. John experienced some temporary continence issues that disappeared within two months and actually experienced an improvement with urinary frequency issues he had before the prostate cancer diagnosis. His erectile dysfunction resolved in two years with the help of Viagra. At ten years post-surgery, John's PSA level remained undetectable, and he continued to be satisfied with his decision to undergo RP.

References

1. Walsh PC, Lepor H. The role of radical prostatectomy in the management of prostatic cancer. *Cancer*. 1987 Aug 1; 60(3 Suppl):526–37.
2. Lepor H, Gregerman M, Crosby R, et al. Precise localization of the autonomic nerves from the pelvic plexus to the corpora cavernosa: A detailed anatomical study of the adult male pelvis. *J Urol*. 1985; 133:207–212.
3. Walsh PC, Lepor H, Eggleston JC. Radical prostatectomy with preservation of sexual function: anatomical and pathological considerations. *Prostate*. 1983;4(5):473–85.
4. Catalona WJ, Carvalhal GF, Mager DE, Smith DS. Potency, continence and complication rates in 1,870 consecutive radical retropubic prostatectomies. *J Urol*. 1999 Aug;162(2):433–8.
5. Walsh PC, Marschke P, Ricker D, Burnett AL. Patient-reported urinary continence and sexual function after anatomic radical prostatectomy. *Urology*. 2000 Jan;55(1):58–61.
6. Rosen RC, Riley A, Wagner G, Osterloh IH, Kirkpatrick J, Mishra A. The international index of erectile function (IIEF): a multidimensional scale for assessment of erectile dysfunction. *Urology*. 1997 Jun;49(6):822–30.

7. Lepor H. A review of surgical techniques for radical prostatectomy. *Rev Urol*. 2005;7 Suppl 2:S11-7.

8. Mirkin JN, Lowrance WT, Feifer AH, Mulhall JP, Eastham JE, Elkin EB. Direct-to-consumer Internet promotion of robotic prostatectomy exhibits varying quality of information. *Health Aff (Millwood)*. 2012 Apr;31(4):760–9.

9. Tosoian JJ, Loeb S. Radical retropubic prostatectomy: comparison of the open and robotic approaches for treatment of prostate cancer. *Rev Urol*. 2012;14(1-2):20–7.

10. Mirheydar HS, Parsons JK. Diffusion of robotics into clinical practice in the United States: process, patient safety, learning curves, and the public health. *World J Urol*. 2012; Epub Dec 29.

11. Williams SB, Chen MH, D'Amico AV, et al. Radical retropubic prostatectomy and robotic-assisted laparoscopic prostatectomy: likelihood of positive surgical margin(s). *Urology*. 2010 Nov;76(5):1097–101.

12. Barry MJ, Gallagher PM, Skinner JS, Fowler FJ Jr. Adverse effects of robotic-assisted laparoscopic versus open retropubic radical prostatectomy among a nationwide random sample of Medicare-age men. *J Clin Oncol*. 2012 Feb 10;30(5):513–8.

13. Schroeck FR, Krupski TL, Sun L, et al. Satisfaction and regret after open retropubic or robot-assisted laparoscopic radical prostatectomy. *Eur Urol*. 2008 Oct;54(4):785–93.

14. Smith JA Jr. Robotically assisted laparoscopic prostatectomy: an assessment of its contemporary role in the surgical management of localized prostate cancer. *Am J Surg*. 2004 Oct;188(4A Suppl):63S–67S.

15. Rosenblum N, Levine MA, Handler T, Lepor H. The role of preoperative epoetin alfa in men undergoing radical retropubic prostatectomy. *J Urol*. 2000 Mar;163(3):829–33.

16. Kowalczyk, Liz. "Mass. cautions hospitals about robotic surgery." *The Boston Globe*. Metro section. March 26, 2013.

17. Rabin, Roni Caryn. "Salesmen in the surgical suite." *The New York Times*. March 26, 2013. p. D1.

18. Sultan R, Slova D, Thiel B, Lepor H. Time to return to work and physical activity following open radical retropubic prostatectomy.

J Urol. 2006 Oct;176(4 Pt 1):1420–3.

19. Diokno AC, Estanol MV, Ibrahim IA, Balasubramaniam M. Prevalence of urinary incontinence in community dwelling men: a cross sectional nationwide epidemiological survey. *Int Urol Nephrol.* 2007;39(1):129–36.

20. Taylor BC, Wilt TJ, Fink HA, et al.; Osteoporotic Fractures in Men (MrOS) Study Research Group. Prevalence, severity, and health correlates of lower urinary tract symptoms among older men: the MrOS study. *Urology.* 2006 Oct;68(4):804–9.

21. Slova D, Lepor H. The short-term and long-term effects of radical prostatectomy on lower urinary tract symptoms. *J Urol.* 2007 Dec;178(6):2397–400; discussion 2400–1.

22. Catalona WJ, Carvalhal GF, Mager DE, Smith DS. Potency, continence and complication rates in 1,870 consecutive radical retropubic prostatectomies. *J Urol.* 1999 Aug;162(2):433–8.

23. McCullough AR, Levine LA, Padma-Nathan H. Return of nocturnal erections and erectile function after bilateral nerve-sparing radical prostatectomy in men treated nightly with sildenafil citrate: subanalysis of a longitudinal randomized double-blind placebo-controlled trial. *J Sex Med.* 2008 Feb;5(2):476–84.

Patient Checklist

If your doctor has recommended radical prostatectomy surgery, bring this checklist with you to your next doctor's visit to get the answers you need to stay healthy.

☐ Will you be doing a nerve-sparing surgery? If not, why? _____
_____
_____

☐ How many prostate cancer surgeries like mine have you done? _____
_____
_____

☐ How soon can I return to work and to regular activities following surgery? _____
_____
_____

☐ How will this surgery impact my urinary control? _____
_____
_____

☐ How will this surgery impact my sexual functioning? _____
_____
_____

☐ After surgery, are there treatments you recommend to help me regain erectile function faster? _____
_____
_____

☐ What is my risk of biochemical recurrence of my cancer? _____
_____
_____

Visit www.sprypubprostate.com to download a printable checklist.

CHAPTER SEVEN

Treatment Choices: Radiation Therapy

One Man's Story

Brian is a 74-year-old retiree and widower who underwent nerve-sparing radical prostatectomy six years ago for a Gleason 7 prostate cancer. The surgery was successful and most of the side effects had disappeared within two years. He still has occasional problems maintaining an erection but doesn't consider this a major issue at this point in time, as he had some ED issues before his prostate cancer diagnosis and had found ways to still enjoy intimacy. Brian religiously attended all follow-up appointments with his doctor and was pleased to have gotten through the cancer treatment experience with relatively few problems.

Four years after surgery, Brian's doctor tells him that the PSA level has risen 0.36 ng/mL. For the past two years, he had calculated Brian's PSA doubling time (PSADT) to be one year. He explains to Brian that these things mean that he may be experiencing what is called a *biochemical recurrence*, or return of his cancer, and orders additional tests. Brian is upset and scared by this news; he tells the doctor that he chose surgery because he thought removal of his prostate guaranteed removal of the cancer.

Brian's doctor is sympathetic and explains that studies have shown that ten years following prostatectomy for prostate cancer, between 15% and 37% of men experience this biochemical recurrence.[1,2,3] This is why they have been following Brian's PSA level so closely; so they can detect any problems early. Based on the negative imaging studies, a prolonged PSADT, and the long time between surgery to BCR, recurrence seems to be localized to a small area in his pelvis, and he is a perfect candidate for salvage radiation treatment.

Radiation Therapy: A Short History

The first reported use of radiation for prostate cancer treatment was in the early twentieth century. Radium, which had been discovered in 1898 by Marie and Pierre Curie, had been used with some success to treat skin cancer shortly after the turn of the century. Physicians in France, Austria, and the United States attempted to harness this success for prostate cancer by placing radium on applicators and inserting them into the urethra and/or rectum of prostate cancer patients.

But the use of radiation for cancer treatment did not really advance significantly until the end of World War II and the development of X-ray beams that could penetrate and deliver radiation to deep tumors without damaging skin and other healthy tissues.[4]

In 1955, physicians at Stanford University introduced the first linear accelerator for clinical use to the United States, and the following year began to use it to administer external beam radiation therapy (EBRT) to prostate cancer patients.[5] In the 1980s, the wide availability of 3-D imaging such as CT scanning led to a new, more effective generation of radiation therapy.

As technology and clinical research advanced, several different types of EBRT were developed. These include intensity-modulated radiation therapy (IMRT), proton beam, and stereotactic body radiation therapy (SBRT), which is often done by a machine called the CyberKnife®. Today, IMRT is the most widely used and available of these therapies for prostate cancer.

Different Types of Radiation Therapy

There are two main categories of radiation therapy for prostate cancer—EBRT and internal radiation therapy (brachytherapy). In EBRT, machines are used to deliver a focused dose of radiation into the prostate cancer. In brachytherapy, small seed-like pellets that contain radioactive material are inserted into the prostate, where they deliver a slow and steady dose of radiation to the cancer.

Will I need hormone therapy after my radiation?

Androgen deprivation therapy (ADT) is often recommended in patients with what we consider to be high-risk disease. The exact duration of ADT is subject to some debate, but in 2013 most would consider a period of two years to be reasonable. Some studies have shown survival advantages with three years of ADT.[6] Usually two years is the minimum for high-risk disease.

Whether or not patients in the intermediate-risk category benefit from androgen deprivation is a subject of debate. In making a recommendation, we look at the individual patient. Where are they on the spectrum of risk? Are they closer to high risk or closer to low risk? Then we look at that profile compared with the patient's medical condition. If patients are older, or they have some history of coronary artery disease, then ADT may do more harm than good. Basically that intermediate-risk group is a grey area where we work with our colleagues to establish and balance disease risk with risk of side effects. Hormone therapy is discussed in detail in chapter 9.

Radiation therapy is usually performed at a hospital or outpatient center by a radiation oncologist. Ideally, the radiation oncologist will work in consultation with a urologist. Again, a treatment approach where doctors share information and collaborate on care planning is the best-case scenario for the patient.

Intensity-Modulated Radiation Therapy

IMRT uses a large machine that actually rotates around the patient, delivering precise doses of radiation from many different angles. It is called *intensity modulated* because the machine is able to deliver beams of varying intensity. The cancer is more precisely targeted with higher-intensity radiation, and healthy tissue is avoided.

When IMRT is used in conjunction with special imaging techniques, it is called *image-guided radiation therapy* (IGRT). IGRT works just like IMRT, except that before each radiation session, a CT scan or other imaging procedure is taken of the prostate. Since the prostate will change size and structure as a result of radiation, this scan gives the radiation oncologist an accurate 3-D view of the prostate to make adjustments in position if needed.

Most patients are fitted for a custom plastic body cradle before treatment begins. This allows the radiation oncologist to put them in the exact same position for treatment at each RT session, resulting in more effective therapy. Each treatment lasts about 15 minutes. IMRT is generally given every day for approximately six weeks, although the length of treatment varies by facility and physician.

Brachytherapy

In brachytherapy, small radioactive pellets, about the size of a grain of rice, are surgically implanted into the prostate (see figure 13). This is done under general anesthesia during a minor outpatient surgery. Before the procedure takes place, the prostate is imaged using ultrasound, CT, or MRI scanning, and a map is created for exact placement of the pellets. About 40 to 100 pellets are typically placed in the prostate.

There are two types of brachytherapy—low-dose rate and high-dose rate. With low-dose rate, the pellets are implanted and left in the body permanently (i.e., there is no surgical removal of them later). With high-dose rate, a radiation source travels into the prostate via guide wires, which are removed after the procedure.

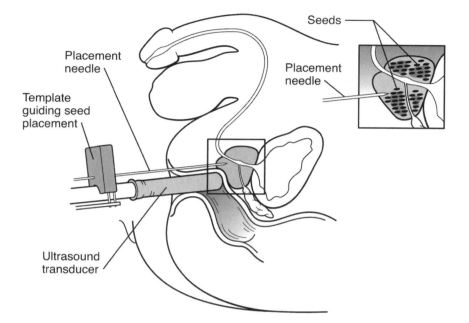

*Figure 13. Brachytherapy seeds within the prostate gland.
Permanent prostate brachytherapy involves placing many
radioactive seeds within the prostate to treat cancer. During the
procedure, an ultrasound probe is placed in the rectum to help guide
the placement of seeds. The seeds, which are typically permanent,
emit radiation that dissipates over a few months.*

The goal of brachytherapy is to very slowly destroy the cancer
while minimizing any damage to surrounding healthy tissue. It is
an effective treatment for men with low-risk prostate cancer confined
to the prostate gland. In intermediate- and high-risk cases, your
treatment team may recommend that brachytherapy is combined with
a course of IMRT and/or hormonal therapy.

My doctor has told me I'm a candidate for prostatectomy surgery or radiation therapy. How do I choose?

Well, first of all, there is no right or wrong answer. The best approach is to find out all the information you can about both. Ask your doctor many questions about how effective each therapy is for your specific cancer and what side effects and complications are to be expected. In our practices, urologists, radiation oncologists, and other specialists work collaboratively so that we can be sure we are providing the most appropriate recommendation for the patient versus just "what we know" in our area of expertise. For younger (age 65 and under) patients, we might suggest surgery first for the simple reason that if cancer recurs later, a patient will have another treatment option with radiation. It is extremely difficult to do radiation first and then try to go back and remove the prostate surgically. So using the surgery option first allows us to use radiation as a safety net treatment later, if required (called *salvage radiation therapy*).

What to Expect after Radiation Therapy

Unlike prostatectomy surgery, where side effects are apparent almost immediately, some complications of radiation therapy actually develop a year or several years following treatment.

Side effects from EBRT may include:

- **Fatigue**—Fatigue is a very common complaint with radiation treatment. This may be partially due to the time demand and stress associated with daily radiation.
- **Bowel Problems**—Toward the end of treatment, men may experience loose stools and irregular bowel movements.
- **Frequent Urination**—Some men experience an increase in urinary frequency during radiation treatment, which usually resolves within a few weeks.
- **Urinary Incontinence**—Incontinence is an uncommon side effect with radiation, but if it does occur, it is usually a year or later following treatment.

- **Urethral Stricture**—The urethra, the tube that carries urine out of the body, may develop scar tissue, and this scar tissue may cause narrowing that interferes with urine flow. This is an extremely rare side effect of EBRT.
- **Erectile Dysfunction**—ED tends to develop between one and three years after radiation treatment is finished. This is likely due to blood vessel changes. Advances in EBRT have improved the odds of overcoming ED over time. One recent study of 1,002 prostate cancer patients found that five years after IMRT treatment, 74% of men who had been fully potent before treatment had regained their sexual function.[7]

Side effects from brachytherapy may include:
- **Migration of Seeds**—The tiny radioactive seeds implanted in brachytherapy may move over time. However, this typically does not cause any health problems.
- **Changes in Urination**—You may have some blood in your urine and pain or burning during urination after the procedure. Longer-term, you may develop problems being able to urinate or you may find yourself having to urinate more often.
- **Bowel Problems**—Due to swelling of the prostate, your bowel habits may change and you may become constipated.
- **Fatigue**—The stress and anxiety of dealing with cancer can wear out patients.
- **Urethral Stricture**—The urethra, the tube that carries urine out of the body, may develop scar tissue, and this scar tissue may cause narrowing.
- **Erectile Dysfunction**—ED is less common with brachytherapy than it is with EBRT. Whether or not a man regains sexual function is largely dependent on his age and level of erectile function prior to treatment.[8]

Men who undergo low-dose brachytherapy may need to limit their exposure to pregnant women, small children, and young animals for a few weeks to a few months following the procedure due to the radiation risk. The duration depends on what isotope is used in the procedure. Usually this just means avoiding lap sitting and long hugs.

Because brachytherapy can make existing urinary symptoms worse, it is usually not recommended for men with substantial lower urinary tract symptoms. Essentially brachytherapy is like lighting a fire in a very small stove, which is effective from a cancer control point of view, but not from a urological point of view. These men may be better off with a course of external beam therapy, which is very gradual and tends to be milder on the urinary system.

Can radiation treatment increase my risk of developing other kinds of cancers?

Some long-term studies have shown an increased incidence of colon, bladder, and rectal cancers in men who have undergone RT for prostate cancer.[9,10,11] So the short answer to the question is yes, but there is an important caveat: the risk is low. A radiation-induced malignancy, if it does occur, has an average latency period of about 15 years. That means they would take 15 years to even begin to develop. With childhood cancers, that's obviously a big concern because patients can live for 60 years longer and they have a lot of time to develop this problem. But in prostate cancer, where many of the men we are treating are 70 and older, the possibility of this happening is extremely low. It's also unlikely in the first place. Most radiologists would estimate the risk of radiation-induced malignancy to be about 0.5%, or one in 200. If we add that many of these patients are being treated in the seventh decade of life, that risk drops even lower.

However, if you are diagnosed earlier in life, you should have a serious discussion with your doctor about your personal risk for developing a secondary cancer after radiation therapy. If you have a life expectancy of 15 years or longer, this may be a factor in your treatment decision.

Is It Right for You?

If cancer has spread beyond the confines of the prostate gland, EBRT is a first-line treatment option. Almost all of these patients would be treated with external beam radiation therapy and hormones. And we often see men who have low- or intermediate-risk disease that is still confined to the prostate, but who feel strongly about not having surgery.

As doctors, our recommendation is driven by an interplay of the patient's medical condition, age, tumor characteristics, and personal preferences. We're looking at the patient's overall health and their other medical problems. We're also looking at what is important to them from a lifestyle perspective. For example, if they have an active sex life and are very concerned about erectile preservation, then brachytherapy may be a more attractive option. Similarly, some patients come in with LUTS, and we would be more likely to recommend EBRT or prostatectomy to them.

Another issue can be time constraints. External radiation is outpatient therapy that requires a commitment to regular daily appointments for several weeks. The practical and logistical issues surrounding the treatment also factor into the decision. On the other hand, brachytherapy is an outpatient surgery that requires less of a time commitment.

Like prostatectomy, radiation therapy is not a guarantee of a cancer cure. Published studies have shown that between 19% and 26% of men who undergo brachytherapy will have a biochemical recurrence of prostate cancer within twelve years.[12] For men treated with EBRT, BCR rates of up to 40% have been reported at seven year follow-up, although some of these results reflect more aggressive cancers.[13]

For this reason, men who undergo radiation therapy need to continue with regular DRE and PSA testing. Normal unirradiated cells in the prostate will continue to produce PSA, although overall PSA levels should start to drop gradually and then level out about two years after treatment.

It's been one year since I had brachytherapy, and my PSA is actually rising, albeit slightly. Does this mean the cancer is returning?

For reasons we don't completely understand, up to 62% of men who undergo brachytherapy for prostate cancer experience a transient rise in PSA called a *PSA bounce*.[14] Sometimes, between one and three years following treatment, the PSA rises 0.2 ng/mL or less and then comes back down to normal levels on its own. Some studies have actually associated PSA bounce with a better overall survival rate for some men.[15,16] If your PSA rise is slight, it may be this bounce phenomenon. Ask your doctor what the numbers mean and if more follow-up testing is warranted.

Emerging Treatments: CyberKnife and Proton Beam

CyberKnife and proton beam therapy are forms of external beam radiation treatment. Both are relatively new radiation options for prostate cancer with a small but growing body of research behind them.

CyberKnife

CyberKnife is a small radiation machine that's mounted on a robotic arm so that it can deliver radiation to different locations with a technique that we call *hypofractionation*. Essentially, it delivers larger doses of radiation so that you end up needing fewer treatment sessions.

Small gold seeds called fiducials must be implanted into the prostate before CyberKnife therapy begins. These serve as markers for the radiation machine. A CT and/or MRI scan and body cradle fitting are also done prior to therapy to ensure the prostate is accurately mapped and the patient is in a fixed position for treatment.

CyberKnife technology is currently FDA approved to treat solid tumors, which include tumors of the prostate. The technology has only been in use since the early 2000s.[17] Initial research is promising; one study reported that 93% of patients undergoing the treatment had no recurrence of their prostate cancer five years post-treatment.[18]

However, we still do not have a lot of long-term data surrounding consistent use, late-stage side effects, and outcomes in prostate cancer treatment. These results may also reflect very early, nonaggressive cancers. Some practitioners are compressing treatments into as few as five treatment sessions, but we don't yet really know the long-term effects of this. As with all new technologies, it's important to separate medical fact from corporate and hospital marketing. More clinical trials are really necessary to establish what the most effective and safe treatment regimen is for CyberKnife patients.

In April 2013, the U.S. FDA issued a voluntary recall notice of the CyberKnife due to issues with some components of the system that affected appropriate targeting of the beam.[19] The manufacturer reported that the recall affected 176 CyberKnife units that would be repaired in the field by technicians.[20]

Proton Beam

Unlike traditional EBRT, which uses X-rays, proton beam radiation therapy uses protons to treat cancerous tissue. Theoretically, these positively charged particles only release their energy when they reach their target, making them less harmful to the healthy tissue they pass through along the way. Protons are also large and less likely to scatter into surrounding tissues and structures after they reach their destination. And unlike some other forms of radiation, they do not exit. You can therefore give a lot of radiation and then it stops on a dime when it reaches the targeted cancer. In theory, this means that you can develop better dose distributions, sparing normal structures around the prostate.

Because of these qualities, proton beam radiation therapy has been in use for more than 40 years in treating tumors, primarily with delicate skull, spinal, and pediatric cancers. But given the significant cost of proton beam therapy equipment (estimates run as high as $200 million), hospitals and healthcare administrators have looked for other ways to monetize their investment. To this end, over the past few decades, researchers have applied proton beam therapy to the high volume business of prostate cancer treatment.

Studies indicate proton beam therapy is similar to brachytherapy and IMRT in terms of cancer control rates.[21,22] And data from several large proton beam therapy centers reported low rates of gastrointestinal, urinary, and sexual side effects.[23] One recent study did find that gastrointestinal toxicity was higher with proton beam therapy.[24] However, no published research to date has demonstrated any significant clinical advantage of proton beam therapy over other EBRT therapies. When you factor in the high cost of treatment, it remains to be seen whether or not proton beam therapy will remain a viable treatment option. More long-term randomized controlled trials are needed.

Again due to cost, proton beam therapy is not widely available, so depending on where you live, you may have limited access to this treatment.

Putting It All Together

After learning more about the IMRT treatments his doctor suggests and meeting with a radiation oncologist, Brian agrees to seven weeks of daily radiation treatment. He quickly finds himself slightly fatigued by the treatment program, but is able to go back and forth to treatment without difficulty. He also finds himself having to get up more often during the night to urinate than he used to during the early weeks of treatment, but his doctor warns him of this possibility before treatment and it starts to lessen as treatment progresses. Other than these temporary issues and some minor gastrointestinal distress, Brian makes it through treatment with no problems.

At a six-month follow-up, Brian's PSA levels are back down to trace amounts. Brian and his doctor agree that if the PSA rises they can discuss treatment options. He has regained most of his energy and has started volunteering at a local cancer center to mentor other men going through prostate cancer treatment.

References

1. Pound CR, Partin AW, Eisenberger MA, et al. Natural history of progression after PSA elevation following radical prostatectomy. *JAMA*. 1999;281:1591–7. PMID: 10235151.

2. Roehl KA, Han M, Ramos CG, et al. Cancer progression and survival rates following anatomical radical retropubic prostatectomy in 3,478 consecutive patients: long-term results. *J Urol*. 2004;172:910–14.

3. Uchio EM, Aslan M, Wells CK, Calderone J, Concato J. Impact of biochemical recurrence in prostate cancer among US veterans. *Arch Intern Med*. 2010;170(15):1390–1395.

4. Slater, James. "From X-Rays to Ion Beams: A Short History of Radiation Therapy." U. Linz (ed.). *Ion Beam Therapy, Biological and Medical Physics*, Biomedical Engineering Springer-Verlag: Berlin. 2012.

5. Bagshaw MA, Hancock SL. "Radiation Therapy of Prostate Cancer at Stanford University: An Experience of 36 Years" Denis, L. (ed.). *Prostate Cancer 2000. ESO Monographs*. Springer: Berlin. 1994. pp. 57–69.

6. Bolla M, Van Tienhoven G, Warde P, et al. External irradiation with or without long-term androgen suppression for prostate cancer with high metastatic risk: 10-year results of an EORTC randomised study. *Lancet Oncol*. 2010 Nov;11(11):1066–73.

7. Spratt DE, Pei X, Yamada J, Kollmeier MA, Cox B, Zelefsky MJ. Long-term survival and toxicity in patients treated with high-dose intensity modulated radiation therapy for localized prostate cancer. *Int J Radiat Oncol Biol Phys*. 2013 Mar 1;85(3):686–92.

8. Snyder KM, Stock RG, Buckstein M, Stone NN. Long-term potency preservation following brachytherapy for prostate cancer. *BJU Int*. 2012 Jul;110(2):221–5.

9. Rapiti E, Fioretta G, Verkooijen HM, et al. Increased risk of colon cancer after external radiation therapy for prostate cancer. *Int J Cancer*. 2008 Sep 1;123(5):1141–5.

10. Sountoulides P, Koletsas N, Kikidakis D, Paschalidis K, Sofikitis N. Secondary malignancies following radiotherapy for prostate cancer.

Ther Adv Urol. 2010 Jun;2(3):119–25.

11. Baxter NN, Tepper JE, Durham SB, Rothenberger DA, Virnig BA. Increased risk of rectal cancer after prostate radiation: a population-based study. *Gastroenterology.* 2005 Apr;128(4):819–24.

12. Potters L, Morgenstern C, Calugara E, et al. 12-Year outcomes following permanent prostate brachytherapy in patients with clinically localized prostate cancer. *J Urol.* 2005;173:1562–6.

13. Khuntia D, Reddy CA, Mahadevan A, Klein EA, Kupelian PA. Recurrence-free survival rates after external-beam radiotherapy for patients with clinical T1–T3 prostate carcinoma in the prostate-specific antigen era. *Cancer.* 2004;100:1283–92.

14. Zelefsky MJ. PSA bounce versus biochemical failure following prostate brachytherapy. *Nat Clin Pract Urol.* 2006 Nov;3(11): 578–9. Review.

15. Hinnen KA, Monninkhof EM, Battermann JJ, van Roermund JG, Frank SJ, van Vulpen M. Prostate specific antigen bounce is related to overall survival in prostate brachytherapy. *Int J Radiat Oncol Biol Phys.* 2012 Feb 1;82(2):883–8.

16. Frank SJ, Levy LB, van Vulpen M, et al. Outcomes after prostate brachytherapy are even better than predicted. *Cancer.* 2012 Feb 1;118(3):839–47.

17. King CR, Lehmann J, Adler JR, Hai J. CyberKnife radiotherapy for localized prostate cancer: rationale and technical feasibility. *Technol Cancer Res Treat.* 2003 Feb;2(1):25–30.

18. Freeman DE, King CR. Stereotactic body radiotherapy for low-risk prostate cancer: five-year outcomes. *Radiation Oncology.* 2011;6(1, article 3).

19. U. S. Food and Drug Administration. Class 2 Recall. CyberKnife System Iris Variable Aperture Collimator Recall number Z-1126-2013. April 16, 2013. [Accessed 5/19/13 at http://www.accessdata.fda.gov/scripts/cdrh/cfdocs/cfRes/res.cfm?ID=116839].

20. Accuray Inc. Accuray Provides Clarification on Recently Initiated Voluntary Recalls. Press Release. April 18, 2013.

21. Coen JJ, Zietman AL, Rossi CJ, et al. Comparison of high-dose proton radiotherapy and brachytherapy in localized prostate cancer: a case-matched analysis. *Int J Radiat Oncol Biol Phys.* 2012 Jan 1;82(1):e25–31.

22. Efstathiou JA, Gray PJ, Zietman AL. Proton beam therapy and localised prostate cancer: current status and controversies. *Br J Cancer.* 2013 Apr 2;108(6):1225–30. doi: 10.1038/bjc.2013.100. Epub 2013 Mar 12.

23. Mendenhall NP, Li Z, Hoppe BS, et al. Early outcomes from three prospective trials of image-guided proton therapy for prostate cancer. *Int J Radiat Oncol Biol Phys.* 2012 Jan 1;82(1):213–21.

24. Sheets NC, Goldin GH, Meyer AM, et al. Intensity-modulated radiation therapy, proton therapy, or conformal radiation therapy and morbidity and disease control in localized prostate cancer. *JAMA.* 2012 Apr 18;307(15):1611–20.

Patient Checklist

If your doctor has recommended radiation therapy, or if you are interested in discussing this option with him, bring this checklist with you to your radiation oncology appointment to get the answers you need to stay healthy.

☐ Am I a candidate for radiation therapy? Why or why not? _____
_____

☐ Are there other treatment options for me outside of radiation? What are they, in order of your recommended preference? _____
_____

☐ What is my risk for developing a secondary cancer after undergoing radiation therapy? _____
_____

☐ If I choose radiation therapy, what type is best for my cancer?
_____

☐ How often will I need to come for treatment? Can you describe a typical appointment? _____
_____

☐ What side effects should I expect from the radiation treatments both during treatment and in the future? _____
_____
_____

☐ What is your personal experience with the form of radiation you are recommending? How long have you been doing it and what kind of success rates have you had? _____
_____

☐ Are there precautions I need to take around my family and friends following treatment? _____
_____

CHAPTER EIGHT

Treatment Choices: Ablation Therapy

One Man's Story

Gary is a 55-year-old sales executive at an insurance company. He leads an active lifestyle, traveling frequently for work and playing in amateur golf competitions every chance he gets. He is engaged to be married to Joanne, a nurse, next month. She has two teenage children from a previous marriage, and Gary is looking forward to being a dad, as he's never had kids of his own.

Three weeks ago, Gary got a phone call from his urologist about elevated PSA results. After discussing his options with his doctor, he underwent an mpMRI and TRUS-guided targeted biopsy, which revealed a Gleason 6 cancer confined to the left lobe of his prostate. Now he is back at the urologist's office learning about his treatment choices. Gary doesn't feel comfortable with the idea of active surveillance due to his young age, but he is alarmed to learn that erectile dysfunction and urinary incontinence are likely side effects of prostate surgery and radiation. As he tells his doctor, he is "not interested in spending his honeymoon playing cards and wearing adult diapers." He agrees to think things over and call back with his decision.

Unhappy with what seems to be a limited offering of treatment options, Gary decides to get a second opinion at the Smilow Comprehensive Prostate Cancer Center at NYULMC, about which Joanne has heard good things. They agree with the pathology results and assessment of his regular urologist. However, they do have one more treatment choice to offer him—mpMRI-guided focal laser ablation to destroy the cancerous tissue, a procedure offered by just a handful of urology/radiology teams in the world. The expertise of Dr. Dan Sperling is solicited as he is an interventional radiologist who has performed the greatest number of MRI-guided laser ablations in the country. The procedure would be done in one day with very well tolerated side effects and few if any lingering complications. In addition, they tell him that his tumor, which is low risk and able to be seen on imaging, is a perfect candidate for the treatment. However, they do advise Gary that the procedure is still a new one, and there is limited short-term and no long-term research on it. He may ultimately require retreatment or radical prostatectomy surgery to control the disease. Despite these caveats, Gary is thrilled at the prospect of destroying the cancer while still maintaining his health and happiness. He schedules the procedure for the following week.

Explaining Ablation: A Minimally Invasive Option

Ablation involves destroying cancerous tissue with extreme temperatures or energy waves. It is less invasive than a prostatectomy surgery because only a very small incision is generally required (and some procedures don't require any incision).

Ablation can either be used to treat the entire prostate gland (called *whole gland ablation*) or to selectively target areas of clinically significant cancers inside the prostate (called *focal ablation*). Energy sources that are approved for use in the United States for tissue ablation include cryoablation and laser ablation. The use of vascular photodynamic therapy and high-intensity focused ultrasound (HIFU) is currently considered investigational in the United States. Independent of the energy source utilized, whole gland ablation is associated with similar risks of radical prostatectomy and radiation therapy. Focal ablation is an exciting new realm of prostate cancer treatment that has great potential for eradicating the aggressive cancer while avoiding incontinence, ED, and other common side effects of traditional prostate cancer treatments.

I don't want surgery or radiation. Is whole gland ablative therapy the answer?

It may be if your cancer is confined to the prostate capsule. However, not all facilities have the expertise and equipment to offer whole gland ablative treatment such as cryotherapy. HIFU is currently not approved in the United States, and whole gland ablation also carries similar risks of urinary and sexual side effects. If you are interested in whole gland cryoablation and it is offered at a treatment facility near you, you should seek out a doctor who is experienced with the treatment. Ideally, you should request outcomes data published in credible medical journals so you can have a realistic expectation of disease control versus complications.

A randomized study conducted in Canada compared whole gland cryoablation to external beam radiation therapy in men with clinically localized disease. The risk of biochemical recurrence was lower in men randomized to whole gland cryoablation.[1] An advantage of cryoablation over radiation therapy is that the treatment is completed in one session. Erectile dysfunction occurs in almost all men undergoing whole gland cryoablation. For older men with significant health problems, aggressive cancers, and ED, cryoablation is a very reasonable option.

Focal Laser Ablation Therapy

In theory, any energy source that ablates tissue can be utilized for focal (or targeted) ablation of the prostate. In order to perform targeted ablation, one needs to accurately identify the target for tissue destruction. Today, MRI is the only imaging technique that reliably identifies the site of clinically significant prostate cancer. Therefore, targeted ablations must be performed using energy sources that are compatible with MRI devices. Laser is the ideal energy source for performing focal therapy of prostate cancers that have been localized to a region of the gland.

Focal laser ablation therapy uses laser energy to heat and destroy cancerous prostate tissue while leaving the surrounding healthy tissue, nerves, and blood vessels untouched. This technology has the potential to control the disease while significantly lowering the risk of incontinence, erectile dysfunction, and other complications associated with surgery and radiation.

Dr. Sperling, one of your authors, is an interventional radiologist who specializes in targeted laser ablation therapy for men with localized prostate cancer. This is an emerging, cutting edge treatment that is truly minimally invasive and can be highly effective. Working in collaboration with a urologist, he uses mpMRI to target areas of clinically significant cancerous tissue and laser technology to destroy it.

A New Paradigm

As discussed elsewhere in this book, regular PSA screening over the past few decades has given rise to a huge increase in the diagnosis of low-risk prostate cancers, which has in turn resulted in significant over-treatment of the disease. Men suffer considerable deterioration of their quality of life when they experience incontinence, erectile dysfunction, and other complications of common prostate cancer treatments such as prostatectomy and radiation. A targeted treatment such as focal laser ablation destroys the cancer while avoiding these critical problems.

The treatment is also unique in that it uses a collaborative approach among healthcare practitioners. Urologists and interventional radiologists work together as a team to diagnose, assess, and treat the cancer. Since a urologist is an expert in diseases of the prostate and urogenital tract and an interventional radiologist is an expert in advanced imaging techniques like mpMRI, this provides you, the patient, with the best of both worlds.

How It Works

Before a focal laser ablation procedure begins, the patient has already undergone mpMRI to determine the exact location and size of the dominant tumor tissue. A targeted biopsy performed in the MRI machine or an ultrasound-guided biopsy using cognitive or computer co-registration establishes the size and aggressiveness of the cancer. These procedures are described in detail in chapter 4.

Today, random biopsies of the prostate are performed to decrease the chance of missing clinically significant disease. The MRI scan creates a detailed prostate map to serve as a blueprint for the ablation procedure. This blueprint also shows the location of sensitive structures like nerves and blood vessels so that your doctor can leave these intact.

The ablation procedure takes place under MRI guidance. The radiologist places a plastic tube into the rectum and guides a very thin laser fiber through this tube and directly into the tumor tissue (see figure 14). Before the procedure begins, the area is numbed with a local anesthetic. Dr. Sperling's technique is unique in that general anesthesia is not required and you will be awake for the procedure.

Once the radiologist and urologist confirm with MRI that the laser fiber is in the central portion of the tumor tissue, the laser is activated to begin slowly heating the tumor to kill the cancer cells. Each area, or lesion, that is created with laser ablation measures approximately 15 mm × 15 mm. For larger tumors, the radiologist will create multiple overlapping laser ablation lesions.

Laser ablation is extremely precise and even lesions located near more sensitive areas, such as the neurovascular bundles and near the urethra, can be safely ablated. The MRI and special software allow precise monitoring of temperature within the tumor and adjacent structures in real time. By using a technology called *MRI thermometry*, the MRI is essentially converted into a virtual thermometer. Small amounts of temperature changes are converted into an image on the ablation software, which allows the doctor to detect how much tissue is destroyed at one time. They can also control the amount of energy transmitted by the laser so that the surrounding healthy tissue and structures aren't harmed.

The whole procedure is typically done in one hour or less. Patients go home about 20 minutes after the procedure, and no urinary catheter

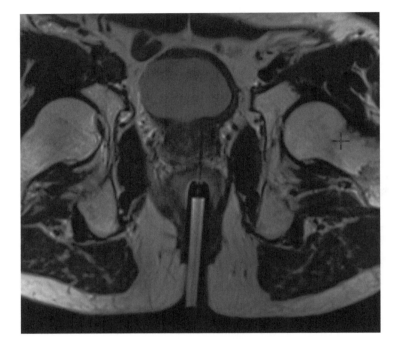

Figure 14. Multiparametric magnetic resonance imaging
showing the thin laser fiber in the tumor tissue.

is usually needed (a catheter may be required in patients who are being treated for a recurrence that have previously undergone other types of therapy).

Pros and Cons

Targeted laser ablation offers an important "safety net" for patients if the tumor is not completely eradicated or new ones develop down the road. Not only can laser ablation be repeated if other prostate cancers develop, but it also preserves the option to later treat men with surgery and radiation if these therapies are ever necessary.

Other benefits of focal laser ablation include:
- **Fast Recovery**—The procedure is minimally invasive, no anesthesia or urinary catheter is required, and men can resume normal activity that evening.
- **Convenience**—It only requires one to two hours in an outpatient facility.
- **Low Risk of Side Effects**—In men who undergo targeted ablation, side effects such as incontinence or erectile dysfunction are extremely rare.[2]
- **High Rates of Apparent Effectiveness**—A recent University of Chicago study found that 78% of patients had no evidence of cancer six months following the procedure.[3]

Because most men start off having multifocal prostate cancer, or cancer in multiple areas of the prostate, those who opt for focal laser ablation may run the risk of "under-treating" the cancer. That is, they may end up with additional cancers requiring treatment later on in other parts of the prostate. The risk of harboring a significant secondary cancer is quite low in regions where the mpMRI is normal and random biopsies failed to identify residual cancer. In addition, it is possible that the laser will not ablate or destroy all of the cancer in the region of interest. And any cancer inadvertently left behind has the potential to metastasize.[4]

Prostate cancer therapies that target the whole gland, such as radical prostatectomy, eliminate all these cancers at once (as long as they have not spread outside of the prostate capsule). Therefore, men electing to pursue targeted ablation must realize there are uncertainties as to whether all the cancer has been eradicated. These men must be followed with routine post-treatment PSA testing, mpMRI, and prostate biopsy. For some, this can be an emotional burden, but for others, it's a good choice that allows them to maintain a high quality of life.

Presumably, regular follow-up screening in men who undergo ablation should catch any residual prostate cancers early on. In addition, these men can go on to have surgery, radiation, or additional targeted ablation procedures later if future testing reveals significant cancer.

Currently, mpMRI-guided focal laser ablation is only available in a handful of facilities in the United States, and very few interventional radiologists are trained in its use. As more long-term clinical studies on its effectiveness in prostate cancer treatment are published, it may become more widely available.

Will focal therapy help me avoid the complications of whole gland ablation?

The biggest advantage of focal therapy is that it leaves surrounding healthy tissue, nerves, and blood vessels untouched. This means that side effects such as erectile dysfunction and incontinence that may occur when the whole gland is treated are virtually always avoided.

Is It Right for You?

If your prostate cancer is not extensive (based on mpMRI, DRE, and prostate biopsy) and considered low or intermediate risk (Gleason 6 or Gleason 7), focal laser ablation may be a good choice for you. For men who are considering active surveillance treatment, ablation can offer a bit more peace of mind without the potentially life-altering side effects of some other prostate cancer treatments.

It is estimated that about 50% of men with low-risk disease based on biopsy actually end up having more aggressive disease. Therefore, we currently understage/undergrade and inappropriately assign about half of the low-risk cancers diagnosed to active surveillance. This is yet another reason why focal ablation may be preferred over active surveillance. It is almost as safe as a biopsy and has the potential to eradicate cancer.

It's important to realize that focal ablation may not be a cure for prostate cancer. While it does destroy cancerous tissue in your prostate, it does not mean you'll never get another tumor. This is why men who undergo targeted ablation need regular follow-up, which is typically regular PSA testing, mpMRI scanning, and interval biopsies. If a new tumor does develop or cancer reappears in the previously ablated area, the laser procedure can be repeated as needed or a radical prostatectomy or radiation can be performed.

I'm really interested in focal laser ablation but my local hospital does not do it. Am I out of luck?

As of the writing of this book, access to this treatment is limited in the United States. Few facilities have both the training and the equipment required to perform mpMRI-guided focal laser ablation for prostate cancer. However, if you are willing to travel, you may be able to find qualified treatment at a major cancer center. Talk to your urologist about your options. Assuming that your health and specific type of prostate cancer make you a candidate for this procedure, he may be able to direct you to a facility that offers it. Appendix A of this book has contact information for Dr. Sperling's center.

Cryotherapy

Cryotherapy for prostate cancer involves freezing the prostate tissue with a gas mixture. The gas is administered through one or more needles inserted through the perineum and into the prostate using transrectal ultrasound guidance. The super-cooled gas forms small ice balls in the prostate. At the same time, warm water is circulated through the urethra to prevent damage to that structure. Traditionally, this treatment has been offered for whole gland ablation in men whose cancer has returned after other treatments such as radiation (known as *salvage treatment*). Cryotherapy has also been advocated as primary treatment for localized prostate cancer. The procedure requires either a spinal block local anesthetic or a general anesthetic and urinary catheterization. Impotency is a common side effect, but incontinence rates following treatment are very low.[5]

Today, cryotherapy is being used along with mpMRI scanning for focal ablation of prostate cancer tumors. By performing cryotherapy in the MRI scanner and using software that provides real-time temperature monitoring, an interventional radiologist delivers an ice ball that surrounds and destroys cancerous tissue in the prostate. This method is not as precise as laser ablation in that there is less control over the size and temperature of the ablation area. But like laser ablation, when performed by an expert this technique has a lower risk of urinary and sexual side effects.[6] Cryotherapy typically requires general anesthesia and an overnight stay in the hospital.

While whole gland cryotherapy has been in wide use since the early 1990s, focal cryotherapy is still in its infancy. Early studies are promising, but the treatment needs more study to determine long-term outcomes for patients.

High-Intensity Focused Ultrasound

High-intensity focused ultrasound (HIFU) is a treatment that uses focused sound waves to destroy prostate tissue. It is the only truly noninvasive treatment for prostate cancer and is administered with an ultrasound probe inserted into the rectum. No needles or incisions are required.

HIFU is being used in both whole gland and focal prostate cancer treatment in many countries outside the United States. The most common side effect with whole gland treatment is urinary retention, an inability to completely empty the bladder that can result in discomfort, frequent bladder infections, and kidney problems. This is usually temporary. Men who undergo HIFU do require urinary catheterization during the procedure and for at least a week afterward. Focal HIFU treatment has been investigated in Europe and appears to have a high success rate with low rates of impotency and urinary side effects.[7]

Both whole gland and focal HIFU treatments are currently only available for prostate cancer treatment outside of the United States. As of mid-2013, HIFU was only approved for investigational use in the United States, and therefore the only way to get this treatment currently is to participate in a clinical trial or to travel outside the United States. It is possible that HIFU will be approved as a salvage treatment following disease recurrence after radiation therapy in the next 18 to 24 months.

Putting It All Together

The morning of his scheduled laser ablation procedure, Gary makes a few last minute business calls and heads for the Sperling Prostate Center. He's given some light sedation to help relax him and a local anesthetic to numb the area where the laser is inserted. Two hours later, he is headed home with virtually no discomfort. That night, he and Joanne celebrate with a candlelight dinner, champagne, and sex. The next day, he's on a plane to visit a client.

At his six-month and one-year follow-ups, Gary's PSA and mpMRI show no evidence of cancer. A TRUS-guided biopsy of the ablated lesion using 3-D co-MRI registration at one year showed no cancer. Today, he and Joanne are celebrating their five-year wedding anniversary and Gary remains healthy, happy, and biopsy cancer free.

References

1. Chin JL, Ng CK, Touma NJ, et al. Randomized trial comparing cryoablation and external beam radiotherapy for T2C-T3B prostate cancer. *Prostate Cancer Prostatic Dis*. 2008;11(1):40–5.
2. Colin P, Mordon S, Nevoux P, et al. Focal laser ablation of prostate cancer: definition, needs, and future. *Adv Urol*. 2012;589160. doi: 10.1155/2012/589160. Epub 2012 May 16.
3. Oto A, Sethi I, Karczmar G, et al. MR Imaging-guided focal laser ablation for prostate cancer: phase I trial. *Radiology*. 2013 Feb 25.
4. Mearini L, Porena M. Pros and cons of focal therapy for localised prostate cancer. *Prostate Cancer*. 2011;2011:584784. doi: 10.1155/2011/584784. Epub 2011 May 10.
5. Babaian RJ, Donnelly B, Bahn D, et al. Best practice statement on cryosurgery for the treatment of localized prostate cancer. *J Urol*. 2008 Nov;180(5):1993–2004.
6. Bahn DK, Silverman P, Lee F Sr, Badalament R, Bahn ED, Rewcastle JC. Focal prostate cryoablation: initial results show cancer control and potency preservation. *J Endourol*. 2006 Sep;20(9):688–92.
7. Muto S, Yoshii T, Saito K, Kamiyama Y, Ide H, Horie S. Focal therapy with high-intensity-focused ultrasound in the treatment of localized prostate cancer. *Jpn J Clin Oncol*. 2008 Mar;38(3):192–9.

Patient Checklist

If your doctor has recommended ablation, or if you are interested in discussing this option with him, bring this checklist with you to your next appointment to get the answers you need to stay healthy.

☐ Am I a candidate for whole gland ablation therapy? If so, what kind do you recommend? If not, why not? _____
_____
_____

☐ Am I a candidate for focal ablation therapy? If so, what kind do you recommend? If not, why not? _____
_____
_____

☐ What side effects should I expect following my ablation procedure? How soon can I resume normal activities? _____
_____
_____

☐ How many ablation procedures have you performed? _____
_____
_____

☐ What follow-up is required after the ablation procedure? What tests will I need and how often? _____
_____
_____

☐ What are the chances of cancer recurring after the ablation procedure? _____
_____
_____

Visit www.sprypubprostate.com to download a printable checklist.

CHAPTER NINE

Treatment Choices: Hormone Therapy

One Man's Story

Jeff is a 53-year-old single man who was diagnosed with a high-risk prostate cancer five years ago. At that time, he had radical prostatectomy surgery. The pathology showed a Gleason 8 cancer with extracapsular extension and positive surgical margins. His lymph nodes were negative for cancer. Jeff's PSA levels had remained very low for the first few years, but are now rising. His PSA was 12 ng/mL and the PSADT, or doubling time, was 4 months. He's also been having some twinges of mild hip pain, which he mentioned to his doctor. His doctor ordered an MRI and bone scan, which revealed that the cancer had recurred and metastasized to the pelvic lymph nodes and a small area of his pelvis.

Right now, Jeff is feeling pretty good. The temporary erectile problems and urinary symptoms he experienced during and after his last prostate cancer treatment resolved long ago. His doctor recommends that Jeff start immediately on a course of androgen deprivation therapy to control the cancer growth. He explains that this isn't a cure, but given Jeff's relatively young age and lack of symptoms, hormone therapy could halt the progression of the disease for several years. He also recommends that Jeff take denosumab (Xgeva) to help prevent skeletal-related events (SREs) like a fracture that could happen in light of his skeletal metastasis. Jeff is also referred to a well-regarded oncologist at a nearby facility for a second opinion and a further discussion of his treatment options.

Androgen Deprivation Therapy

Hormone therapy is also known as androgen deprivation therapy (ADT). Androgens are the male hormones such as testosterone and dihydrotestosterone. While there is no evidence that higher levels of androgens are associated with a greater incidence of prostate cancer, we do know that they can fuel a cancer's growth if present. So ADT is designed to slow cancer growth by either lowering levels of these hormones in the body or preventing androgens from affecting cancer cells.

ADT is most appropriate for men with cancers that have metastasized to bone or other visceral sites. Some men with high-grade disease and rapidly rising PSADTs are presumed to have metastasis even if they are not seen on imaging studies. In this setting, ADT is often initiated. It is not a cure, but it can shrink and slow the growth of prostate tumors even after the cancers have spread to distant sites in the body and control the disease for many years.

How It Works

There are a few different types of ADT. These therapies may be used alone, in combination, or as a companion to radiation treatment. They include surgical castration, drugs that lower androgen production by the body, and drugs that alter the way the body uses androgens.

One of the earliest treatments for prostate cancer was *surgical castration*, or removal of the testicles (also known as *orchiectomy*). Dr. Charles Huggins received the 1966 Nobel Prize in Medicine for discovering that orchiectomy or medical castration with estrogens causes dramatic regression of metastatic prostate cancer.[1] Because the testicles produce an estimated 90% of a man's testosterone, it was an effective way to halt cancer growth. Surgical castration is still an option today, but few men choose it because there are other equally effective, noninvasive hormone treatment options.

Luteinizing hormone-releasing hormone (LHRH) agonists or analogs are drugs that significantly lower the amount of testosterone produced by the testicles. These drugs are also called gonadotropin-releasing hormone (GnRH) agonists. When LHRH agonist therapy starts, testosterone levels may actually go up temporarily, a phenomenon known as "tumor flare," before they begin to decrease. LHRH agonists used in the United States include leuprolide (Lupron, Eligard), goserelin (Zoladex), triptorelin (Trelstar), and histrelin (Vantas). These drugs are injected by your doctor. Depending on which one you take, you may need to get them monthly, several times a year, or annually.

There is also a class of drugs known as LHRH antagonists that, like the agonists, work to suppress testosterone production in the testicles. However, these drugs work faster and they do not cause the tumor flare that is characteristic of the agonists. Drugs in this class are sometimes called gonadotropin-releasing hormone (GnRH) receptor antagonists, and include degarelix (Firmagon) and abarelix (Plenaxis). The limitation of LHRH antagonists today is the lack of long-term depot formulations, so monthly injections are required.

Antiandrogens are drugs that prevent the body from processing androgens. These drugs are taken by mouth and are usually used as an adjunct, or companion, treatment to other hormone therapies like LHRH agonists or antagonists. This is because, by themselves, they are typically not as effective as these other treatment options. Antiandrogen drugs include bicalutamide (Casodex), flutamide (Eulexin), and nilutamide (Nilandron). When taken alone, the antiandrogens can cause painful and permanent gynecomastia, or breast tissue enlargement.

I have prostate cancer and low testosterone ... is it safe to replace testosterone?

This is controversial because, as we said, prostate cancers are fueled by testosterone. And for late-stage cancers, the answer to this question is definitely no. But there are an increasing number of men who have been treated successfully for early prostate cancer who by all criteria appear to be cured. A few years following treatment these men may experience erectile problems or other significant symptoms of hypogonadism (low testosterone) and may benefit from testosterone supplementation.

An increasing number of urologists, oncologists, and internists are becoming more open to initiating testosterone therapy in these patients when they feel absolutely confident that the patient's prostate cancer has been cured and that the quality of life of this patient would be significantly enhanced with testosterone replacement therapy. It is important to realize that low testosterone causes a variety of troubling problems, including osteoporosis, fatigue, hot flashes, elevated lipids, depression, and muscle wasting. Testosterone replacement will likely reverse these problems. Still, testosterone therapy should be undertaken only in a cooperative dialogue with the patient and his doctors, and these patients should be closely monitored while on testosterone replacement therapy.

Pros and Cons

Surgical castration is the least expensive hormone therapy option with known efficacy. But due to its permanency and invasiveness, men may shy away from that choice.

All androgen deprivation essentially throws a man into the equivalent of a menopausal state. These are the same types of symptoms you might see in men with low testosterone. They will have drops in their libido, they'll have sweating, they'll have weight gain. Potential side effects of ADT include:

- hot flashes

- impotence and/or loss of libido
- breast tenderness and/or tissue growth
- loss of muscle mass
- weight gain
- fatigue
- mental fog and/or memory loss
- depression
- anemia
- decrease in HDL (good) cholesterol

There is also a risk of more serious side effects in some men who take LHRH agonists (GnRH agonists), including cardiovascular disease, diabetes, and osteoporosis. To avoid these issues, men on ADT may undergo regular heart, metabolic, and bone density testing.[2]

Men who take antiandrogens in combination with LHRH drugs commonly experience diarrhea. These men should also have regular liver enzyme tests, as antiandrogens can affect liver function.

Are there any ways to decrease the side effects of hormone therapy?

Relief is possible for some of the side effects of hormone therapy. For example, antidepressant drugs often help with hot flashes, as well as lifting symptoms of depression. Regular exercise can help men on ADT regain muscle and bone mass and lose extra weight, as well as also helping with depression and fatigue. And there are also several drugs available to help treat any osteoporosis that results from hormone treatment.

When It Stops Working

Hormone therapy is a mainstay treatment approach for many men with metastatic disease. But as time goes on, the majority of men become resistant to the hormone treatment. This is because cancer evolves through genetic instability as it becomes more advanced. Eventually, some cancer cells may be able to grow without needing testosterone, and as these cells multiply, ADT becomes ineffective. In other cases, the cancer cell manufactures testosterone. When this happens, cancer is said to be hormone resistant or hormone refractory.

Hormonal therapy is no longer controlling my disease, what's next?

If the hormone therapy you are using stops working, your doctor may switch hormones or try another secondary hormone therapy to see if that is effective. If your prostate cancer continues to advance, chemotherapy is usually the next step.

Secondary Hormonal Therapy

If your prostate cancer becomes resistant to first-line ADT treatment, there are secondary hormonal treatments your doctor may recommend. These may be prescribed when first-line hormones fail or following a course of chemotherapy. These include:

- **Abiraterone acetate (Zytiga)**—This drug stops the production of androgens in other non-testicular tissues, including the adrenal glands, the small glands located on the kidneys, which secrete 10% of the body's total androgen production. It also halts androgen production in the tumor tissue itself. Zytiga is prescribed with prednisone to lessen side effects, which include joint and muscle pain. Other common side effects include fluid buildup and low blood potassium levels. When abiraterone is administered to men with castrate-resistant prostate cancer after chemotherapy, abiraterone can increase life expectancy a median of 4.6 months when compared to placebo.[3] Recent studies have also shown that abiraterone decreases time to development of metastasis when prescribed to men with asymptomatic castrate-resistant prostate cancer prior to chemotherapy.[4]
- **Enzalutamide (Xtandi)**—A newer drug that prevents the body from processing androgens, it is currently only approved for use in men with castrate-resistant prostate cancer after

chemotherapy. Side effects from this medication include diarrhea, dizziness, and fatigue. A small percentage of men will develop seizures and experience an increased incidence of falls. Similar to abiraterone, the median increase in life expectancy can be 4.8 months.[5]

Beyond Hormones

Eventually, all late-stage prostate cancers become resistant to existing primary and secondary hormone therapies. But in the past decade, very exciting and viable chemotherapy and immunotherapy options have become available for patients.

Chemotherapy drugs target and damage the structure of prostate cancer cells. It is typically a late-stage treatment because it has significant side effects, including hair loss, mouth sores, vomiting and nausea, diarrhea, loss of appetite, anemia, and a weakened immune system. The first-line chemotherapy agent is usually docetaxel (Taxotere), which is given with prednisone. There are a number of other chemotherapy drugs available if Taxotere is ineffective.

Prostate cancer metastasized to bones can be extremely painful. Now we also have medications that are reducing the ability of these tumor cells to stimulate bone resorption, or the process by which bone breaks down. When this process is accelerated, as can happen in metastatic prostate cancer, bone is destroyed more quickly than it is replaced and fractures and other troublesome skeletal problems are often the result. Medications to address this problem include drugs such as zoledronic acid (Zometa) and denosumab (Xgeva). These play very valuable roles in preserving a better quality of life for patients with prostate cancer that has become metastatic to bone.

Finally, a new immunotherapy, or cancer vaccine, called sipuleucel-T (Provenge) was approved for U.S. men with asymptomatic metastatic hormone refractory prostate cancer in 2010. This treatment is unique in that it uses a man's own white blood cells to create an immune system cocktail that targets and kills cancer cells. While again not a cure for cancer, Provenge has been shown to extend life in clinical trials.[6] Researchers are now looking at whether or not immunotherapy may be beneficial earlier in the disease process.

Putting It All Together

Jeff visits the new oncologist for a second opinion for painful skeletal metastasis from his prostate cancer. That physician also recommends androgen deprivation therapy, so Jeff consents to a regimen of ADT and Xgeva injections every four weeks. He also comes in for regular blood tests to monitor his overall health.

One year after starting hormones, Jeff's PSA has dropped dramatically and bone and CT scans show his tumor has totally regressed. He has experienced hot flashes and erectile and libido problems that are normal side effects of ADT, as well as some temporary weight gain. He was able to manage the weight gain, however, by keeping up with daily swimming, an exercise he enjoys. He's also noticed that this has helped with his mood. Jeff's oncologist recommends they stay the course with his current treatment and he agrees.

References

1. "Charles B. Huggins–Nobel Lecture: Endocrine-Induced Regression of Cancers." Nobelprize.org. [Accessed May 19, 2013]. http://www.nobelprize.org/nobel_prizes/medicine/laureates/1966/huggins-lecture.html]

2. U.S. Food & Drug Administration. FDA Drug Safety Communication: Update to Ongoing Safety Review of GnRH Agonists and Notification to Manufacturers of GnRH Agonists to Add New Safety Information to Labeling Regarding Increased Risk of Diabetes and Certain Cardiovascular Diseases. October 20, 2010. http://www.fda.gov/Drugs/DrugSafety/ucm229986.htm.

3. De Bono JS, Logothetis CJ, Molina A, et al. Abiraterone and increased survival in metastatic prostate cancer. *N Engl J Med.* 2011;364:(21):1995–2005.

4. Ryan CJ, Smith MR, Molina A, et al. Interim analysis (IA) results of COU-AA-302, a randomized, phase 3 study of abiraterone acetate (AA) in chemotherapy-naïve patients (pts) with metastatic castration-resistant prostate cancer (mCRPC). ASCO 2012; p7.

5. Xtandi [prescribing information]. Northbrook, IL: Astellas Pharma US, Inc.; 2012.

6. Kantoff PW, Higano CS, Shore ND, et al.; IMPACT Study Investigators. Sipuleucel-T immunotherapy for castration-resistant prostate cancer. *N Engl J Med.* 2010 Jul 29;363(5):411–22.

Patient Checklist

If your doctor has recommended hormone therapy, bring this checklist with you to your next doctor's visit to get the answers you need to stay healthy.

☐ What hormone treatment do you recommend for my particular prostate cancer and why? _____
_____
_____
_____

☐ What side effects should I expect? _____
_____
_____
_____

☐ What can I do to manage side effects? _____
_____
_____
_____

☐ How often and how will I get the hormone? _____
_____
_____
_____

☐ Is hormone therapy my only treatment choice? _____
_____
_____
_____

☐ How will we monitor for growth of my cancer? _____
_____
_____
_____

Visit www.sprypubprostate.com to download a printable checklist.

CHAPTER TEN

Living beyond Cancer: Life after Treatment

One Man's Story

Two years ago, just after his 48th birthday, Stan found out he had prostate cancer. He was in good health at the time, with no real complaints except for a lack of sleep due to shift changes in his job. His doctor found a nodule during a routine DRE, which started Stan on a journey of tests, scans, and biopsies that revealed a Gleason 7 tumor. One month later, Stan was checking in to the hospital for radical nerve-sparing prostatectomy surgery.

After the surgery, Stan was told that the tumor margins were clear. It appeared as though the prostate, and the cancer within it, was removed successfully. He experienced some discomfort after the surgery, had a catheter in his penis for a week, and had incontinence for six weeks. But Stan was warned of these temporary side effects ahead of time, knew what to expect, and was therefore emotionally and physically prepared to handle them.

Stan was also told about possible ED. As part of a penile rehabilitation program, he was started on a daily dose of Viagra shortly after surgery in order to prevent penile smooth muscle atrophy while the nerves innervating the penis regenerated. His doctor also suggested he periodically use a vacuum pump for increasing blood flow to the penis and restoring an erect penis adequate but not ideal for sexual intercourse. Stan's wife Mary came to his first postsurgical doctor's appointment with him and they took in all this together.

Will It Come Back?

The transition from prostate cancer patient to prostate cancer survivor can be a difficult one for some men. Even if all detected cancer was removed or eradicated through treatment, there is always the fear that it may return or spread. It is natural to experience some level of anxiety around this, and it's not unfounded. Statistically, biochemical recurrence, a rise in PSA levels that may indicate the presence of active prostate cancer, is not uncommon. This is why regular follow-up with your doctor after treatment is complete is so important.

Biochemical recurrence varies by the type of treatment you received. For men who have radical prostatectomy surgery, BCR is defined by a PSA of >0.2 ng/mL measured on at least two occasions. For those who have undergone radiation therapy as a first-line treatment, the criteria is a bit different. The professional organization for radiation oncologists, the American Society for Therapeutic Radiology and Oncology (ASTRO), defines BCR as a 2 ng/mL or higher rise above the nadir PSA (or lowest level it has reached post-treatment).[1]

If you meet the criteria for BCR, it means that active cancer is likely, either within the prostate or outside of it. However, it is not proof positive that cancer has recurred. Further testing, including imaging studies, is often obtained. If a prostatectomy is being considered after failed RT (called *salvage prostatectomy*), a biopsy of the prostate must be performed to confirm local disease. Biopsies are generally not performed when there is a BCR after RP since it is rarely positive. This is because BCR after RP is often detected very early by the rising PSA, when cancer is microscopic and random core biopsies are likely to miss it.

What Now? Regular Follow-Up

Your doctor should review your follow-up plan with you at your first post-treatment appointment. The recommendation will vary by physician and patient profile. But for most men with non-metastatic cancer who have had their cancer removed or destroyed through surgical, radiation, or ablative treatment, follow-up will be every six months for at least five years. You will have regular PSA tests to catch any recurrence early. Your doctor may also recommend periodic imaging tests such as MRI following focal ablation.

If you have metastatic prostate cancer, your treatment will be ongoing and focused on containing further spread of the cancer and managing any unpleasant symptoms you are experiencing. You should remain an active participant in your treatment plan. When your doctor recommends changes, ask why and make sure you are fully informed on what side effects you may experience. Keep a written record of symptom changes that you can share with your doctor at each visit. Stay involved and encourage your significant other to do so as well.

When should I stop getting a PSA test?

As previously mentioned, regular PSA testing after treatment is important in catching any cancer recurrence early. The level of change in PSA between tests is typically more critical than the actual PSA value by itself, so monitoring this on a regular basis remains important. But if you are of an advanced age or have significant co-existing health problems and have had undetectable PSA levels for decades, at some point your doctor may suggest PSA testing is not required. As always, talk to your doctor about your specific health needs.

If you haven't already, now is a good time to get all of your medical records in order. If at any point in the future you need to see a new doctor, having a full set of records related to your cancer-related treatment history is important. These should include:

- **Pathology Reports**—Request a copy of all biopsy and surgical pathology reports.
- **Imaging Reports**—Request a digital copy (e.g., CD, DVD) of all scans from the imaging facility or radiologist's office.

- **Operative Reports**—If you have had a radical prostatectomy, request a copy of the surgical report from your surgeon or hospital.
- **Radiation Reports**—If you have had radiation therapy, request a treatment summary from your radiation oncologist.
- **Hormone or Other Drug Treatment**—Keep a list of all cancer-related medications you have taken and are currently taking, including dosage and special instructions. Note the dates you started and discontinued a medication.
- **Hospital Discharge Summary**—If you had inpatient prostate cancer treatment, keep a copy of the summary you received at discharge.

If you do need to pass these records along to a new physician at any point, make sure you keep a copy for your own files.

Staying Emotionally Healthy

Cancer is a life-threatening and, subsequently, a life-changing condition. For many men, going through cancer treatment offers a good opportunity to reassess life priorities, a time to reflect on where they've been and rethink where they are headed. If we must find a silver lining in cancer, which is certainly a terrible disease for anyone to have to deal with, it is this unique opportunity to really look at your value system and see what really matters to you—family, career, lifestyle, etc. You may find that things that used to aggravate or upset you really don't bother you much anymore with your new post-cancer perspective on life.

Dealing with Side Effects

Urinary, sexual, and bowel-related side effects of treatment are troublesome to many men. As you know by now, these will often improve with time, patience, and, in some cases, additional treatment.

Being well informed about what is "normal" following treatment, and being prepared to cope with it, is the best way to get through this sometimes-difficult post-treatment period. You may need to make temporary changes in your schedule and activities to deal with some issues. For example, if your work or recreational activities involve a lot of travel or outdoor time, you may need to change your routine to have closer access to bathroom facilities.

Remember, prostate cancer and recovery affect other people in your life, too. Make sure your spouse or significant other is also aware of the side effects with which you are dealing. Having their emotional support can be extremely helpful during your recovery.

My penis is shorter since my prostate cancer surgery. No one ever told me this could happen. I'm angry and upset. How could this happen?

A small percentage of men experience some minor and temporary shortening of the penis following prostatectomy or radiation therapy.[2] This is caused by nerve or blood vessel damage in the penis. One study found that men lose up to one centimeter of penile length following radical prostatectomy. The good news is that most men recover this length within two years of surgery and have regained their pre-surgery length at four-year follow-up.[3]

As far as being upset with your doctor, this is a natural reaction. Yes, most urologists will and should mention this potential side effect as you discuss treatment options. However, realize that most physicians do their best to make patients aware of all the potential side effects from cancer treatment and are not trying to hide any information from you. In addition, because cancer treatment is never a simple procedure and there are a wide array of potential outcomes, hospitals and practitioners require patients to read and sign a consent form that lists all these complications—from the rarest to the most common—in great detail. We encourage you to approach your doctor with your concern constructively. Tell him you wish you had known about this possibility early on and would like to discuss what you can do to address the problem now. Penile rehabilitation, discussed elsewhere in this book, may be helpful in speeding the process of recovering penile length.

Transitioning to Cancer Survivor

Most men experience some level of anxiety at prostate cancer diagnosis and throughout treatment. There is fear of the unknown and a constant parade of doctor's appointments, laboratory tests, and hospital visits that can disrupt life for weeks and months. Once you've passed the milestone of your last treatment session, it can be tough to return to your "regular" pre-cancer life of work, home, and family and let go of all of the worry and fear. You may also be anxious about the cancer coming back or spreading and your vulnerability to other health problems.

In some cases, this persistent anxiety is linked to depression and poor sexual performance.[4] Anxiety may be inhibiting the return of sexual function, or erectile problems may be feeding your anxiety. Either way, support groups and/or therapy may be helpful if you find that anxiety and depression are getting in the way of daily functioning and enjoyment of life. If depression is ongoing and persistent, there are medications that may help.

Intimacy and Sex after Treatment

It's important to have realistic expectations about sex following prostate cancer treatment. The goal should be to try and return erectile function to the level it was at before treatment. Depending on your age and health, this may have been limited to begin with, and you should not expect your erections to be better than they were before diagnosis.

All men should have a healthy dose of patience. It is not uncommon for men to continue to recover erectile function up to several years following treatment. Give yourself time.

One issue men may experience that often doesn't come up in discussion with their doctor before treatment is incontinence during sex. Men may leak urine during foreplay or sexual activity. While this can be awkward for you and your partner, just knowing it is a possibility ahead of time can alleviate any anxiety. This problem may be easily remedied by urinating before any sexual contact.

Is erectile dysfunction treatable?

Absolutely. There are several medications and devices that can help you regain your erections. Younger men and men who were able to get healthy erections before undergoing cancer treatment are more likely to regain their potency post-treatment. Drugs called PDE-5 inhibitors (e.g., Viagra, Levitra, Cialis), penile injections, and vacuum pumps are all designed to facilitate blood flow to the penis. Time seems to be the most important factor in recovering erectile function; you may see improvements as long as three years out from surgery. Chapter 6 has more advice on dealing with ED side effects.

After radiation, radical prostatectomy, or whole gland ablation of the prostate, the discharge of semen is eliminated. In some men a small discharge of sticky fluid will appear just prior to orgasm. This fluid is from the urethral glands and contains no sperm.

Even if you aren't able to maintain an erection hard enough for penetration and intercourse, there are still plenty of other ways to achieve intimacy and pleasure with your partner. Erection is not necessary for orgasm, and with a loving partner whom you trust, you may find that your sex life is more adventuresome than ever.

Healthy Habits

Maintaining a healthy lifestyle, with plenty of exercise, nutritious food, and other healthy habits, grows in importance as you age. Men with other health conditions, such as high blood pressure, diabetes, or heart disease, should focus on staying on top of those treatments. If you still smoke, quitting is the single best thing you can do to improve your health, reduce your risk of cancer recurrence, and prevent osteoporosis if you are on ADT.

Other than seeing my doctor for regular follow-up, are there other things I can do to prevent my cancer from coming back?

There are no specific drugs, interventions, or lifestyle changes that are clinically proven to prevent cancer recurrence. But it is a great idea to try to maintain a healthy lifestyle, which is likely to promote a healthy immune system. And that means achieving a healthy body weight, making certain you get restorative sleep, and making certain that the nutrient value of your food is rich enough so that you can enhance your immunity. Chapter 1 has more tips for maintaining your prostate health.

If you have brothers or an adult son, make sure they are aware of their increased risk for developing prostate cancer. They should talk to their own doctor or urologist about their specific risk profile and the screening schedule that's right for them.

Putting It All Together

Stan recovers his continence fairly quickly, and within a month after treatment he no longer needs incontinence pads. He and his wife also start to ease back into intimacy. After three months, Stan begins to have morning erections, which his doctor tells him are a good sign of recovery. Stan and Mary are close and communicative, and they find new ways to express their intimacy. Eight months after surgery, he is able to achieve an erection with a vacuum pump and maintain it for intercourse. Two years post-treatment, he has returned to almost the same level of erectile function that he was at before his cancer diagnosis with the use of Cialis.

Stan has now had three consecutive PSA tests with results of 0.0 ng/dL. He is comfortable with his doctor's assurance that he has an excellent prognosis and is likely cured. With his recovery of sexual function and the good PSA results, his anxiety level significantly drops, and he and Mary begin making plans for a trip to Europe that they have been dreaming about for years.

References

1. Roach M 3rd, Hanks G, Thames H Jr, et al. Defining biochemical failure following radiotherapy with or without hormonal therapy in men with clinically localized prostate cancer: recommendations of the RTOG-ASTRO Phoenix Consensus Conference. *Int J Radiat Oncol Biol Phys.* 2006 Jul 15;65(4):965–74.

2. Parekh A, Chen MH, Hoffman KE, et al. Reduced penile size and treatment regret in men with recurrent prostate cancer after surgery, radiotherapy plus androgen deprivation, or radiotherapy alone. *Urology.* 2013 Jan;81(1):130–4.

3. Vasconcelos JS, Figueiredo RT, Nascimento FL, Damião R, da Silva EA. The natural history of penile length after radical prostatectomy: a long-term prospective study. *Urology.* 2012 Dec;80(6):1293–6.

4. Tavlarides AM, Ames SC, Diehl NN, Joseph RW, Castle EP, Thiel DD, Broderick GA, Parker AS. Evaluation of the association of prostate cancer-specific anxiety with sexual function, depression and cancer aggressiveness in men 1 year following surgical treatment for localized prostate cancer. *Psychooncology.* 2013 Jun;22(6):1328–35. doi: 10.1002/pon.3138. Epub 2012 Aug 1.

Patient Checklist

Bring this checklist with you to your first post-treatment doctor's visit to get the answers you need to stay healthy.

☐ How often should I be coming back for follow-up care? How many years will follow-up care last? _____
_____
_____
_____

☐ What will follow-up care consist of? _____
_____
_____
_____

☐ Should I be starting penile rehabilitation? _____
_____
_____
_____

☐ Are there any treatments or strategies to lessen my urinary symptoms? _____
_____
_____
_____

☐ Are there any symptoms that should be red flags for me to come in for an appointment? _____
_____
_____
_____

Visit www.sprypubprostate.com to download a printable checklist.

Information and Support Resources for Men with Prostate Cancer

Medicine and healthcare are constantly evolving. To keep current on the latest advances in prostate cancer detection and treatment, visit

Smilow Comprehensive Prostate Cancer Center
www.prostate-cancer.med.nyu.edu
and
NYU Langone Medical Center
www.NYULMC.org/menshealth

Sperling Prostate Center
www.sperlingprostatecenter.com
1-877-60-LASER (1-877-605-2737)
Learn about mpMRI-guided prostate cancer detection and focal laser treatment, and find out if treatment is available in your area.

Many organizations provide valuable support for patients and families. We've included a list of some key groups, but others to meet specific patient needs can be found online.

Alliance for Prostate Cancer Prevention (APCaP)
www.apcap.org
The APCaP promotes prostate cancer awareness, education, and advocacy. Special emphasis is directed toward prostate cancer prevention strategies for healthy men in their 40s and 50s.

American Cancer Society (ACS)
www.cancer.org
1-800-227-2345
Information and support for a prostate cancer diagnosis from the American Cancer Society. "Man to Man," a community-based ACS program, connects men with other prostate cancer survivors via monthly support meetings.

CancerCare
www.cancercare.org
1-800-813-HOPE (1-800-813-4673)
Free, professional support services for anyone affected by cancer. Talk to an oncology counselor, get connected with a support group, or find financial help and resources.

MaleCare
www.malecare.org
1-212-673-4920
A volunteer men's cancer support group and advocacy national nonprofit organization with prostate cancer support groups, newly diagnosed cancer support groups, advanced prostate cancer, men diagnosed under age 50, and gay cancer survivor support groups throughout the United States.

National Cancer Institute
www.cancer.gov/prostate
1-800-4-CANCER (1-800-422-6237)
English and Spanish language information on prostate cancer statistics, prevention, screening, diagnosis, and treatment from the National Cancer Institute, part of the National Institutes of Health. Includes information on clinical trials for prostate cancer patients.

Patient Advocates for Advanced Cancer Treatments
www.paactusa.org
1-616-453-1477
PAACT raises prostate cancer awareness, providing patients with treatment options and more.

Prostate Cancer Foundation
www.pcf.org
1-800-757-CURE (1-800-757-2873)
A nonprofit organization dedicated to curing prostate cancer by
directing funds to the most promising clinical research. Their website
offers a wealth of information on the latest developments in prostate
cancer detection and treatment.

Prostate Cancer Research Institute
www.prostate-cancer.org
1-310-743-2110
Supports research and disseminating information that educates and
empowers patients, families, and the medical community.

The Prostate Cancer Roundtable
www.prostatecancerroundtable.net/
Acts as a forum through which all members of the U.S. prostate
cancer advocacy community can act in concert to ensure a shared set
of legislative and scientific priorities that affect the prevention,
detection of risk, diagnosis, and management of prostate cancer.

Prostate Conditions Education Council
www.prostateconditions.org
The organization focuses on saving and improving the lives of men
and their loved ones through early detection, research, education,
and awareness for prostate cancer and all prostate conditions.

Prostate Health Education Network, Inc. (PHEN)
www.prostatehealthed.org
1-866-456-PROSTATE (1-866-456-7767)
Focuses on eliminating the disparity in African American prostate
cancer detection and mortality rates. PHEN's mission also includes
advocacy efforts to increase the overall support and resources to
wage a war on prostate cancer that will eventually lead to a cure for
the disease for the benefit of all men.

The Prostate Net
www.prostate.net
Website for men's health, wellness, nutrition and lifestyle with a focus on prostate and related disorders.

The Urology Care Foundation
www.urologyhealth.org
1-800-828-7866
The official foundation of the American Urological Association. Use their site to find out more about prostate cancer or find a urologist in your area.

Us TOO International Prostate Cancer Education and Support Network
www.ustoo.com
1-800-80-UsTOO (1-800-808-7866)
This grassroots organization offers more than 300 peer-to-peer support groups across America, as well as education programs for patients and their loved ones.

Zero: The Project to End Prostate Cancer
www.zerocancer.org
1-888-245-9455
Zero is working toward a day when there will be zero prostate cancer deaths and diagnoses. They fund cure-based research through local and national events and grants and conduct free prostate cancer screening programs.

Abbreviations Used in This Book

5-ARI drugs 5-alpha-reductase-inhibitor drugs
ACP American College of Physicians
ADT androgen deprivation therapy
ART adjuvant radiation therapy
ASAP atypical small acinar proliferation
ASTRO American Society for Therapeutic Radiology and Oncology
AUA American Urological Association
BCR biochemical recurrence
BPH benign prostatic hyperplasia
CT computerized tomography
DRE digital rectal examination
EBRT external beam radiation therapy
ECG electocardiogram
ED erectile dysfunction
ERSPC European Randomized Study of Screening for
     Prostate Cancer
FDA Food and Drug Administration (U.S.)
GnRH gonadotropin-releasing hormone
GPS genomic prostate score
HGPIN high-grade prostatic intraepithelial neoplasia
HIFU high-intensity focused ultrasound
IIEF International Index of Erectile Function
IGRT image-guided radiation therapy

IMRT intensity-modulated radiation therapy
LHRH luteinizing hormone-releasing hormones
LUTS lower urinary tract symptoms
mpMRI multiparametric magnetic resonance imaging
MRI magnetic resonance imaging
NCCN National Comprehensive Cancer Network
NSAIDs nonsteroidal anti-inflammatory drugs
NYULMC New York University Langone Medical Center
PCA3 prostate cancer gene 3
phi Prostate Health Index
PLCO Prostate, Lung, Colorectal, and Ovarian
PSA prostate-specific antigen
PSAD PSA density
PSADT PSA doubling time
PSAV PSA velocity
RALRP robotic-assisted laparoscopic radical prostatectomy
RP radical prostatectomy
RPP radical perineal prostatectomy
RRP radical retropubic prostatectomy
SBRT stereotactic body radiation therapy
TRUS transrectal ultrasound
USPSTF U.S. Preventive Services Task Force
UTI urinary tract infection

Acknowledgments

Sincere thanks and gratitude to my mentor Dr. Patrick C. Walsh, University Distinguished Service Professor of Urology at Johns Hopkins University, who inspired my interest in prostate cancer, guided my academic career, instilled in me to critically question what is known and search for the truth, and above all that the patient always comes first. To the thousands of men with prostate cancer who over the past 27 years sought my expertise, judgment, and guidance and through these interactions and experiences taught me the art of medicine and healing. —HL

The authors would like to thank our colleague Dr. Nicholas Sanfilippo, Assistant Professor of Radiation Oncology at the NYU School of Medicine and member of the Smilow Comprehensive Prostate Cancer Center, for his expert contributions and input to the radiation therapy portion of this book.

A special thanks also to Paula Ford-Martin, an award-winning health and general interest writer, who was invaluable in taking all of our words and thoughts and creating a cohesive text for the patient.

Index

Illustrations are indicated by **bold** page numbers.

Index

Index

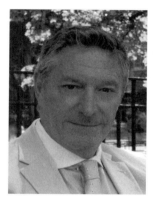

Steven Lamm, MD, is the director of the Men's Health Center at New York University Medical Center and a practicing internist. He is well-known as the house doctor on ABC-TV's *The View*, regularly offering his analysis and commentary on television and radio programs, including *Today*, *Oprah*, *Nightline*, *Dateline*, and *Fox News*. Dr. Lamm has published extensively on a variety of medical topics. His best-selling books include *No Guts, No Glory* (2012) and *Thinner at Last* (2005).

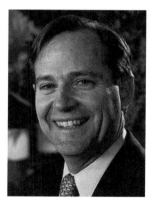

Herbert Lepor, MD, is one of the leading experts in the field of prostate cancer. He is currently the Martin Spatz Chairman of the Department of Urology and the Director of the Smilow Comprehensive Prostate Cancer Center at the NYU Langone Medical Center in New York. He was previously appointed Chairman of Urology at NYU School of Medicine at the age of 37, the youngest chairman of a major academic urology department in the country at that time. Dr. Lepor has written more than 300 articles on the topic of prostate cancer in peer-reviewed academic publications. He has made important contributions to the screening, detection, and treatment of prostate cancer.

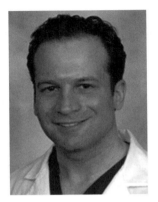 **Dan Sperling**, MD, DABR, is the Medical Director at the Sperling Prostate Center, New York, NY. A leading specialist in the diagnosis and treatment of prostate tumors through magnetic resonance imaging and laser ablation procedures, Dr. Sperling is certified by the American Board of Radiology and licensed in New York and New Jersey.